CARNIVORE DIET

FOR

LONGEVITY & VITALITY

Unlock the Secrets to Optimal Health, Mental Clarity, and Emotional Wellness

Julianna Irvin Saladino

Julianna Irvin Saladino

CARNIVORE DIET FOR LONGEVITY & VITALITY

Unlock the Secrets to Optimal Health, Mental Clarity, and Emotional Wellness

Copyright 2024

TABLE OF CONTENT

- Stress Resilience and Coping Mechanisms: How this diet influences emotional stability.
- Boosting Self-Confidence Through Diet: Feeling empowered by improved health.

Chapter 3: Nutritional Myths & Misconceptions

Cholesterol and Heart Health

- The Cholesterol Debate: Why cholesterol isn't the villain.
- LDL, HDL, and Triglycerides Explained: Understanding your bloodwork.
- Real Heart Health Markers: What really matters when assessing heart disease risk.

Fiber and Gut Health

- The Role of Fiber—Necessary or Overrated?
- How the Gut Adapts to a Carnivore Diet: Short-term adjustments and long-term benefits.
- Microbiome Health Without Plants: A look at bacteria and gut flora in meat-eaters.

Sustainability and Ethical Considerations

- Is a Meat-Only Diet Environmentally Friendly?
- Humane Sourcing and Ethical Eating: Choosing responsibly sourced meat.
- Addressing Ethical Concerns for Vegans and Vegetarians: A balanced discussion.

Chapter 4: Customizing the Carnivore Diet

Variations of the Carnivore Diet

- Strict Carnivore vs. Carnivore Adjacent: Different approaches to the diet
- Adding Minimal Plants or Dairy: Flexibility within the carnivore framework.
- The Zero-Carb Approach: Who benefits from cutting out carbs entirely.

Adjusting for Lifestyle

- The Busy Professional's Plan: Quick and easy meals for those on the go.
- Fitness Enthusiast's Carnivore: Enhancing athletic performance with protein.
- Family-Friendly Carnivore Meals: How to feed your family while following the diet.

Dietary Challenges and Adjustments

- Overcoming Sugar Cravings: How to handle the toughest part of transitioning.
- Dealing with Social Situations: Navigating dining out and events.
- Tailoring the Diet for Specific Health Conditions: From autoimmune issues to metabolic disorders.

Chapter 5: Carnivore Diet & Longevity

Anti-Aging Benefits

- The Role of Protein in Preserving Muscle Mass

- Collagen and Skin Health: Why carnivores may have a youthful glow.

- Bone Health and Longevity: Strong bones through meat and marrow.

Preventing Chronic Disease

- Reversing Insulin Resistance: A deep dive into metabolic health.

- Heart Disease Prevention: The real impact of a carnivore diet on cardiovascular health.

- Cancer and the Carnivore Diet: Examining the evidence for anti-cancer properties.

Cognitive and Neurological Longevity

- Protecting Brain Health as You Age

- Alzheimer's and Diet: The carnivore connection to brain diseases.

- Enhancing Cognitive Function in Later Years: Real-life stories of mental agility.

Chapter 6: The Emotional Journey of the Carnivore Diet

Emotional Benefits

- Stabilizing Mood Swings: How cutting carbs reduces emotional volatility.

- Food and Happiness Correlation: Emotional upliftment through dietary choices.

- Building Confidence in Your Choices: How empowerment comes from aligning health with goals.

Coping with Criticism and Skepticism

- Dealing with Naysayers and Skeptics: Responding to critics in social settings.

- Trusting Your Body's Signals: Learning to rely on personal experience over external opinions.

- Maintaining Motivation on Tough Days: Strategies for staying committed to the diet.

Community and Support

- Finding Like-Minded People: Where to connect with fellow carnivores.

- Online and Local Support Groups: The role of social support in diet success.

- Inspiring Others with Your Journey: Sharing your progress and influencing change.

Chapter 7: Carnivore Diet Recipes & Meal Plans

Essentials for Your Pantry

- Must-Have Ingredients for the Carnivore Kitchen

- Preparing Proteins Like a Pro: Cooking tips for various meats.

- Quick, Simple Carnivore Snacks: Easy-to-make, nutrient-packed meals.

Daily Meal Plans

- 7-Day Beginner Meal Plan: Easy-to-follow steps for new adopters.

- Advanced Meal Plan for Long-Term Success: More variety and complexity for seasoned carnivores.

- Meals for Special Occasions: Staying carnivore while celebrating.

Delicious and Creative Carnivore Recipes

- Breakfast Options: Protein-packed start to the day.

- Hearty Lunch and Dinner Ideas: Main meals to satisfy cravings.

- Indulgent Treats and Drinks: Ways to indulge within the carnivore framework.

Chapter 8: Sustaining Long-Term Success

Measuring Long-Term Health Markers

- Tracking Blood Work and Biometrics: What to watch for.

- Longevity Studies and Insights: How carnivore dieters fare long-term.

- Adjusting the Diet Over Time: When and how to modify based on your changing needs.

Dealing with Plateaus

- Why Plateaus Happen: Understanding the body's adaptation process.

- Breaking Through Plateaus: Strategies to reignite fat loss or muscle gain.

- Staying Motivated Long-Term: Tapping into deeper purpose and commitment.

Final Words on Lifestyle Integration

- Balancing Carnivore with Other Life Goals: Career, family, and beyond.

- Building a Sustainable, Enjoyable Routine

- Embracing a Lifelong Journey: How to make the carnivore diet a sustainable and fulfilling part of your life.

AUTHOR'S FINAL NOTE

ABOUT THE AUTHOR

CHAPTER 1

The Carnivore Diet Unveiled

The carnivore diet, which centers exclusively on animal products, has been gaining traction in recent years as a potential solution for everything from weight loss to mental clarity. However, this way of eating is not a modern fad. In fact, it's deeply rooted in the evolution of human diets. To understand why this diet has resurged in popularity, we must first look at its origins, explore the modern transformations, and debunk the misconceptions that often surround it.

Origins and History

Ancestral Eating Patterns

When we consider the history of human eating habits, we find that for the majority of our existence, humans relied heavily on animal-based nutrition. Our early ancestors were hunter-gatherers, and their survival depended largely on their ability to hunt animals. Archaeological evidence supports the notion that meat, fat, and organs from animals provided the bulk of our ancestral diet, particularly during periods when plant-based foods were scarce.

In contrast to the modern world, where agriculture and the domestication of plants play a significant role, early humans had no such conveniences. Instead, they thrived in a world where the availability of plant foods was seasonal, limited by geography, and often inconsistent. Hunting large game like mammoths, elk, and other herbivores was not only necessary for survival, but an efficient way to fuel the human body. Animal-based diets were rich in essential nutrients that promote brain development, sustained energy, and provided the necessary building blocks for growth. In fact, some scientists argue that our shift to a diet heavy in animal protein and fat contributed directly to the evolution of our large brains.

Anthropologist Miki Ben-Dor, in his research, suggests that around 2 million years ago, early humans became "hyper-carnivores," subsisting mainly on meat. This period coincided with a reduction in tooth size, indicating that early humans were adapting to a more meat-heavy diet. These evolutionary traits suggest that the human body has been optimized for nutrient-dense, meat-based eating over millennia.

While hunting was critical to our survival, it wasn't just about the meat. Every part of the animal was consumed — from muscle and fat to organs, bones, and marrow. These provided essential vitamins, minerals, and fatty acids that plants alone couldn't offer. The liver, for example, is a rich source of vitamin A, and bone marrow provides high-quality fats essential for energy. This all-encompassing consumption of the animal played a crucial role in sustaining life, fueling our ancestors through harsh climates, demanding physical challenges, and long migrations.

Modern Adaptations

As civilization progressed, agriculture and the cultivation of grains began to take hold. Around 10,000 years ago, the dawn of farming brought a significant shift in the human diet. Grains, legumes, and other plant-based foods became staples for many societies, leading to what some call the "Neolithic Revolution." However, despite this shift, it wasn't until much more recently that plant-based eating became synonymous with health. In fact, for thousands of years, the elite and warrior classes in many societies continued to rely on meat as their primary source of sustenance, while plant foods were often seen as food for the poor.

The carnivore diet, in its modern form, is a return to this ancestral way of eating, but it has adapted to contemporary needs and knowledge. Over the past few decades, the rise of low-carb diets like Atkins and keto has paved the way for carnivorism. Where keto limits carbs to a minimum and allows for some plant-based foods, the carnivore diet takes things further by eliminating them entirely, focusing only on animal products such as meat, eggs, and dairy (in some versions).

So, why has the carnivore diet gained such a foothold in the wellness world today? Much of its popularity stems from anecdotal success stories. Individuals have reported drastic improvements in their health—ranging from weight loss and reduced inflammation to better mental clarity and mood stabilization. In many cases, these are people who have struggled with autoimmune diseases, gut disorders, or mental health issues, often after trying a myriad of diets that didn't deliver lasting results.

Shawn Baker, a former orthopedic surgeon and one of the most prominent figures in the carnivore movement, has championed the diet after experiencing his own health transformation. In his book, The Carnivore Diet, he emphasizes the benefits of eliminating plant-based foods that might trigger inflammation or sensitivities in some individuals. Many who follow Baker's approach have shared stories of reversing conditions like Crohn's disease, eczema, and even depression by shifting to an all-meat regimen.

Scientifically, while much of the research on carnivorism is still emerging, some studies support the potential benefits of reducing carbohydrates and plant-based anti-nutrients (such as lectins, phytates, and oxalates), which can interfere with mineral absorption or cause gut irritation in some individuals. Dr. Paul Saladino, another advocate for carnivore diets, highlights in his work that removing plants entirely allows the body to heal and thrive without the potential side effects caused by plant-based toxins.

However, while these modern adaptations of the carnivore diet cater to an individual's health and lifestyle choices, they still honor the evolutionary biology that has shaped human physiology for millennia. It is this combination of ancestral wisdom and modern health benefits that makes the carnivore diet an intriguing approach for many seeking optimal health.

Common Misconceptions

Despite its rise in popularity, the carnivore diet faces its share of skepticism and misconceptions. One of the most persistent myths is that a meat-based diet is inherently bad for cardiovascular health. The conventional wisdom for decades has been that saturated fat, which is prevalent in animal products, leads to heart disease by raising cholesterol levels. However, the scientific understanding of fat, cholesterol, and heart disease has evolved.

Recent studies have shown that saturated fat may not be the primary villain it was once thought to be. A 2010 meta-analysis published in the *American Journal of Clinical Nutrition* found no significant evidence to conclude that dietary saturated fat is associated with an increased risk of coronary heart disease. Furthermore, emerging research highlights that it's not total cholesterol or LDL (low-density lipoprotein) that drives heart disease risk, but rather the size and density of LDL particles. Small, dense LDL particles (which are more likely to result from a diet high in processed carbohydrates and sugars) are far more dangerous than the larger, fluffier particles often found in those following low-carb, high-fat diets like carnivore.

Another common misconception is that without plant-based foods, people on the carnivore diet will miss out on essential nutrients like fiber, vitamins, and antioxidants. While it's true that plants provide fiber, proponents of the carnivore diet argue that fiber may not be necessary for digestive health after all. Some studies, including a 2012 paper in the *World Journal of Gastroenterology*, suggest that reducing or eliminating fiber can improve certain gastrointestinal symptoms, like bloating and constipation. Furthermore, carnivore diet advocates point to the bioavailability of nutrients in animal products. Nutrients such as vitamin B12, iron, and zinc are more easily absorbed from animal sources than from plants, meaning that a well-planned carnivore diet can meet nutritional needs without supplementation.

One of the more contentious debates surrounding the carnivore diet is the question of sustainability. Critics argue that meat-heavy diets contribute to environmental degradation and are unsustainable in a world facing climate change. However, this issue is more nuanced than it appears. Studies have shown that regenerative farming practices, which focus on rotational grazing and restoring soil health, can help mitigate the environmental impact of livestock farming. Moreover, the carnivore diet emphasizes quality over quantity—prioritizing ethically raised, pasture-fed, and sustainably sourced meats.

Lastly, there is the misconception that the carnivore diet is too extreme, unsustainable, or difficult to maintain long-term. While it may seem restrictive to eliminate entire food groups, many who follow this diet report finding it surprisingly easy to stick to. Without the blood sugar swings caused by carbohydrates and the constant need to snack, many carnivore dieters feel fuller for longer periods, leading to less frequent cravings and more consistent energy throughout the day.

Conclusion

The carnivore diet represents a return to our ancestral roots, aligning modern science with evolutionary biology. While it may challenge conventional dietary norms, its rising popularity speaks to its potential to address chronic health issues in a simple, effective way. Understanding the historical context, the modern adaptations, and clearing up common misconceptions is essential for anyone considering this approach. As we uncover more research and listen to individual stories, the carnivore diet is emerging not just as a trend but as a viable path toward optimal health, mental clarity, and emotional well-being.

The Carnivore Diet Unveiled

In recent years, the carnivore diet has drawn attention not only for its historical and ancestral significance, but for the science that underpins its effectiveness. To truly understand how the diet works, it's crucial to delve into its macronutrient composition, the process of ketosis, and the superior bioavailability of animal-based nutrients. These elements work together to create a powerful system that fuels the body, supports optimal health, and addresses some of the common challenges we face with modern diets.

Understanding the Science Behind It

The carnivore diet, at its core, is built on three pillars: high-quality protein, beneficial fats, and minimal to zero carbohydrates. This macronutrient breakdown is what makes it unique and effective for many who adopt it. But how exactly do these elements contribute to the overall benefits people experience on this diet?

Macronutrient Breakdown

In a typical carnivore diet, most of the calories come from two primary sources: protein and fat. These macronutrients are essential not only for survival but for optimal functioning of the body.

Carbohydrates, which are the focus of most modern diets, are almost entirely eliminated, and this shift dramatically changes how the body operates.

Protein is the building block of life. It plays an essential role in repairing tissues, maintaining muscle mass, producing enzymes and hormones, and supporting immune function. For those following a carnivore diet, the bulk of their protein intake comes from high-quality sources such as beef, lamb, pork, poultry, and fish. These animal proteins contain all the essential amino acids in the right proportions, making them a complete source of protein. This is a significant advantage over plant-based proteins, which often lack one or more essential amino acids, forcing those who avoid animal products to combine various foods to meet their nutritional needs.

For many people who adopt the carnivore diet, protein intake is often higher than on traditional diets. And there's a reason for this. Studies have shown that high-protein diets support muscle retention, especially during weight loss, and promote feelings of fullness, which can naturally reduce calorie intake. This satiety effect is particularly beneficial for those who struggle with cravings and overeating on high-carb diets. Additionally, protein has a higher thermic effect of food (TEF) compared to fats and carbohydrates, meaning the body burns more calories digesting protein than it does with other macronutrients.

While protein takes center stage, fat plays an equally critical role in the carnivore diet. Unlike the typical low-fat diets promoted in the past, the carnivore diet embraces fat as a vital energy source. Healthy fats from animal sources—such as saturated fat, monounsaturated fat, and omega-3 fatty acids—fuel the body's energy needs in the absence of carbohydrates. These fats not only provide sustained energy but also support brain function, hormone production, and the absorption of fat-soluble vitamins (A, D, E, and K).

One of the fascinating aspects of the carnivore diet is how the body adjusts to running primarily on fats rather than carbohydrates. For those transitioning from a typical high-carb diet, this switch can feel daunting at first. However, the body is highly adaptable, and once it shifts into a fat-burning mode, many people report feeling more energized, focused, and less reliant on constant meals or snacks.

The Role of Ketosis

One of the central mechanisms that explains the success of the carnivore diet is ketosis. Ketosis occurs when the body burns fat for energy instead of carbohydrates. When carbohydrate intake is restricted, as it is on the carnivore diet, the body's glycogen stores (which are essentially stored carbohydrates) become depleted. Once those stores are exhausted, the body begins to break down fats into molecules called ketones, which are then used for fuel.

This metabolic state of ketosis can have a profound impact on both physical and mental health. For one, burning fat as the primary energy source tends to provide more consistent energy levels throughout the day, as there are no drastic spikes and crashes in blood sugar, which are common on a carbohydrate-heavy diet. This stability is one reason why many people on the carnivore diet report increased mental clarity, focus, and productivity. Without the constant rollercoaster of blood sugar fluctuations, brain function becomes more stable, leading to sharper cognitive abilities and fewer instances of "brain fog."

Moreover, ketosis has been shown to have other health benefits beyond just energy management. Research suggests that ketones are a more efficient fuel source for the brain, which is why ketogenic diets are often used as therapeutic treatments for neurological disorders like epilepsy. A study published in the *journal Frontiers in Aging Neuroscience* even posits that ketones may help protect the brain against age-related diseases like Alzheimer's by reducing oxidative stress and inflammation. This cognitive benefit is why many carnivore diet proponents, like Dr. Paul Saladino, claim that the mental clarity experienced on the diet is one of its most powerful effects.

Ketosis is also linked to fat loss, as the body becomes more efficient at mobilizing and using stored fat as an energy source. This fat-burning process is a cornerstone of why many people experience rapid weight loss when they first adopt the carnivore diet, especially if they've been consuming a high-carb diet beforehand. Additionally, ketosis has a positive effect on insulin sensitivity, which is crucial for managing and preventing metabolic diseases such as type 2 diabetes. By keeping insulin levels low and steady, the carnivore diet allows the body to regulate blood sugar more effectively, reducing the risk of insulin resistance—a key factor in many chronic health issues.

Bioavailability of Nutrients

While the macronutrient composition and ketosis are vital to understanding the success of the carnivore diet, there's another critical factor that sets it apart from other diets: the bioavailability of nutrients. Bioavailability refers to how efficiently the body can absorb and utilize nutrients from the foods we eat. On a carnivore diet, where the focus is solely on animal-based foods, nutrient bioavailability is maximized.

Animal-based foods contain all the essential vitamins and minerals the body needs in highly bioavailable forms. For example, the iron found in meat, known as heme iron, is far more easily absorbed by the body than non-heme iron found in plants. This distinction is especially important for individuals who are at risk of iron deficiency or anemia, as the bioavailability of heme iron can drastically improve iron levels without the need for supplementation.

Similarly, vitamin B12, an essential nutrient for brain function and energy production, is found exclusively in animal products. Deficiency in this vitamin can lead to fatigue, cognitive decline, and nerve damage, all of which can be prevented with adequate intake from meat, eggs, and organ meats. The superior bioavailability of vitamin B12 in animal-based foods ensures that those following a carnivore diet are less likely to experience deficiencies compared to those on plant-based diets, which often require B12 supplementation.

Another nutrient worth mentioning is vitamin A, which plays a crucial role in maintaining healthy vision, skin, and immune function. While some plant-based foods, like carrots, contain beta-carotene (a precursor to vitamin A), the body must convert it into the active form of vitamin A (retinol) to use it effectively. Unfortunately, this conversion process is not very efficient, and factors like genetics and overall health can reduce the body's ability to make the conversion. Animal sources, such as liver, provide vitamin A in its preformed, bioavailable form, which can be readily used by the body.

Beyond vitamins, animal-based fats are also more bioavailable than plant-based oils. For example, the omega-3 fatty acids found in fatty fish like salmon and mackerel are far more readily utilized by the body than the omega-3s found in plant sources like flaxseed. This is because the animal-based omega-3s (EPA and DHA) are in the forms the body needs, while plant-based omega-3s (ALA) must first be converted, and this conversion is often inefficient.

The same goes for minerals. Zinc, calcium, and magnesium are all present in bioavailable forms in animal products, whereas plant foods often contain compounds like phytates and oxalates, which can bind to these minerals and inhibit their absorption. This is a key reason why proponents of the carnivore diet argue that animal-based nutrition is superior for overall health. The body can efficiently extract and use the nutrients it needs without the interference of anti-nutrients found in many plant-based foods.

Conclusion

The science behind the carnivore diet is rooted in its optimal macronutrient composition, the metabolic benefits of ketosis, and the superior bioavailability of nutrients from animal-based foods. This combination not only fuels the body more efficiently but also addresses many of the nutritional deficiencies and metabolic challenges that plague modern diets. By understanding how these elements work together, it becomes clear why the carnivore diet can offer such profound health benefits for those who adopt it. As more research emerges, it is becoming increasingly evident that this way of eating is not just a return to ancestral patterns, but a scientifically grounded approach to achieving optimal health.

The Carnivore Diet Unveiled

The carnivore diet, though simple in concept, requires more than just a shift in what you eat—it demands a mental, emotional, and practical transformation. To embark on this journey successfully, you need to address common psychological barriers, understand the key foods that will fuel your body, and equip yourself with the right tools to track your progress. Making such a significant change may feel overwhelming, but with the right mindset, preparation, and strategies in place, the carnivore diet can lead to transformative results.

Getting Started

Transitioning to a new way of eating, especially one as distinct as the carnivore diet, is not just a physical challenge but a mental one. The first step in any major lifestyle shift is preparing yourself mentally and emotionally for the journey ahead.

Preparing Mentally for the Shift

Adopting the carnivore diet can feel daunting, particularly if you've spent years or decades following conventional dietary advice that emphasizes variety, plant-based foods, and avoiding fats. One of the most common psychological barriers people face when considering the carnivore diet is the fear of eliminating such a large portion of their existing diet. The thought of cutting out all fruits, vegetables, grains, and even snacks can seem extreme. But overcoming this mental hurdle is key to success.

One way to mentally prepare is by reframing the diet as a return to simplicity rather than a restriction. Instead of focusing on what you can't have, think about what you're adding to your life: high-quality, nutrient-dense food that nourishes your body in ways processed and plant-based foods may not. The carnivore diet is a celebration of simplicity, returning to the basics of human nutrition and allowing your body to function in its most natural state.

For many, the initial skepticism about eliminating carbohydrates can be a major obstacle. After all, we've been told for decades that we need carbs for energy. However, countless individuals who have made the switch to carnivore report feeling more energetic and clear-headed without the constant ups and downs that accompany a carb-heavy diet. Research supports this, showing that fat and protein are more efficient and consistent energy sources than carbohydrates. By focusing on the potential improvements in energy, mental clarity, and overall health, it becomes easier to commit to the shift.

Another mental challenge comes from social situations. Food is deeply ingrained in our social fabric, and it can be difficult to navigate family gatherings, holidays, or dinners with friends when your diet is so different. One approach is to communicate your reasons for adopting the carnivore diet in a clear, positive way, focusing on the benefits you expect to gain. Instead of explaining what you're cutting out, talk about how this shift supports your goals for better health and well-being. This positive framing can help others understand your decision and potentially even support you.

Finally, be prepared for the mental challenge of breaking habits and cravings. Many people find that the first few weeks of the carnivore diet are the most challenging, as their body adjusts to the lack of sugar and refined carbohydrates. Cravings for bread, sweets, and even fruits may surface, but it's important to remember that these cravings are temporary. Over time, as your body adapts, those cravings will fade, and many people report losing their taste for sugary and processed foods altogether. Embrace this adjustment period as part of the process, knowing that on the other side lies better energy, mood stabilization, and improved health.

Key Foods to Include
Once you're mentally prepared, the next step is understanding what you'll actually be eating on the carnivore diet. At first glance, the diet may seem limited, but in reality, it offers a wide variety of nutrient-dense foods that can be tailored to your preferences and needs. The foundation of the carnivore diet is simple: high-quality proteins, healthy fats, and nutrient-rich organs.

The primary focus should be on quality animal proteins, such as beef, pork, lamb, chicken, turkey, and fish. Red meat, particularly from grass-fed sources, is especially rich in essential vitamins and minerals like iron, zinc, and B vitamins. Fatty cuts of meat are preferred on the carnivore diet because they provide the energy your body needs in the absence of carbohydrates. Ribeye steaks, fatty ground beef, pork belly, and lamb chops are all excellent choices that combine high-quality protein with satiating fats.

For those who are more adventurous or want to maximize their nutrient intake, organ meats are an incredibly valuable addition to the diet. Foods like liver, kidney, heart, and bone marrow are packed with vitamins and minerals that are hard to find in other foods. Liver, for example, is one of the most nutrient-dense foods on the planet, providing high levels of vitamin A, B12, folate, and iron in a form that is easily absorbed by the body. For those new to organ meats, starting with small amounts or incorporating them into ground meat dishes can make them more palatable.

Fats are a critical component of the carnivore diet, both for energy and to support the absorption of fat-soluble vitamins. Don't be afraid to embrace animal fats like tallow, lard, and butter. These fats are not only essential for energy but also help keep you full and satisfied. If you're eating leaner cuts of meat, adding fats like butter or ghee can ensure you're meeting your body's energy needs.

Seafood is another excellent option for those following the carnivore diet, particularly fatty fish like salmon, mackerel, and sardines, which are rich in omega-3 fatty acids. These essential fats are crucial for brain health, inflammation control, and heart health. Shellfish like oysters and shrimp also provide a wealth of nutrients like iodine, selenium, and zinc.

While the focus is on meat and animal products, many carnivore dieters also include eggs and dairy, depending on their tolerance. Eggs are a perfect balance of protein and fat, and they're versatile enough to be a staple for many on the diet. Dairy, especially in its full-fat forms like cream, cheese, and yogurt, can be included, but some people find that they need to limit or avoid it due to sensitivities or digestive issues.

The key to succeeding with the carnivore diet is to find a variety of foods that you enjoy and that provide the nutrients your body needs. By focusing on whole, unprocessed animal products, you can ensure that you're getting high-quality protein, fats, and essential vitamins and minerals without the anti-nutrients and inflammatory compounds often found in plant-based foods.

Tools for Tracking Progress

Starting the carnivore diet is a significant shift, and tracking your progress is crucial to staying on track and ensuring long-term success. Luckily, there are several tools and strategies available to help you monitor your journey and make adjustments as needed.

One of the simplest yet most effective tools is keeping a food journal. This doesn't need to be a complex or time-consuming task—just a place to record what you eat each day, how you feel, and any changes you notice in your body or energy levels. Tracking your meals can help you spot patterns, such as which foods make you feel the best or when cravings tend to strike. A journal can also help you stay accountable and focused, especially in the early days of the diet when temptation might be high. Beyond just tracking what you eat, make note of your mood, digestion, sleep quality, and any physical changes. This holistic approach can provide valuable insights into how your body is adjusting and what areas might need more attention.

For those who prefer digital tools, there are several apps available that can help you track your carnivore diet journey. Apps like MyFitnessPal and Chronometer allow you to log your meals, track macronutrients, and even monitor your micronutrient intake to ensure you're hitting all your targets. While you don't necessarily need to track calories on a carnivore diet, some people find it helpful, especially in the beginning, to ensure they're eating enough fat to sustain energy levels. Monitoring your protein and fat ratios can also help you tweak your meals for optimal performance.

Another useful tool is regular blood testing to track changes in your health markers over time. Many carnivore dieters find that their cholesterol levels, triglycerides, and markers of inflammation improve significantly after making the switch. By working with a healthcare provider, you can monitor these markers to ensure the diet is benefiting your health. Blood tests can also help track micronutrient levels, such as vitamin D, B12, and iron, which can further validate the success of your dietary changes.

For those who are interested in tracking body composition, devices like bioimpedance scales or even simple tape measurements can be useful. While weight loss is not the primary goal for everyone on the carnivore diet, many people experience a reduction in body fat and an increase in muscle mass. By taking regular measurements of your waist, hips, and other areas, you can track physical changes even if the number on the scale doesn't move as much as you expect.

Perhaps most importantly, pay attention to how you feel. While numbers and data are helpful, the true measure of success on the carnivore diet comes from your day-to-day experience. Are you feeling more energized, focused, and satisfied? Has your digestion improved? Are you experiencing fewer cravings and better control over your eating habits? These subjective experiences are often the best indicators that the diet is working for you.

Conclusion

Getting started with the carnivore diet requires not just a shift in what you eat, but also a mental and emotional commitment to the process. By preparing yourself mentally for the change, focusing on nutrient-dense animal products, and using tools to track your progress, you can navigate the transition with confidence. The carnivore diet, while simple in its approach, offers a powerful path to better health, and with the right mindset and strategies in place, it can lead to profound physical and mental transformations.

CHAPTER 2

Health Benefits of the Carnivore Diet

The carnivore diet, as extreme as it may seem at first glance, has been quietly revolutionizing the lives of countless individuals. Far from being just another trend, this diet has the potential to profoundly reshape one's health—physically, mentally, and emotionally. While the idea of consuming only animal-based products may still be met with skepticism in some circles, those who commit to this way of eating often experience remarkable improvements that extend far beyond weight loss. This chapter will delve deeply into the various health benefits of the carnivore diet, supported by scientific research and personal stories, to illuminate the true potential of this dietary approach.

Physical Health Improvements

The first and most obvious benefits of the carnivore diet are physical. From metabolic shifts to better energy levels and improved digestion, this way of eating can offer a transformative experience for many.

Weight Loss and Metabolism Boost

One of the most talked-about benefits of the carnivore diet is its potential to facilitate weight loss while preserving muscle mass. But what makes this diet particularly effective for those seeking to shed body fat while maintaining lean muscle?

At the heart of the carnivore diet is a dramatic reduction in carbohydrate intake, often leading the body to enter a state known as ketosis. In ketosis, the body shifts from burning carbohydrates for energy to burning fat. This shift can lead to significant fat loss, especially for those who have struggled with diets high in refined carbs and sugars. But it's not just about burning fat—it's also about maintaining muscle, which is critical for long-term health and metabolism.

Protein, a cornerstone of the carnivore diet, plays a crucial role in muscle preservation. High-protein diets have been shown to help maintain lean muscle mass even in calorie-restricted states. Research has demonstrated that diets rich in protein not only help build and preserve muscle but also boost the metabolism. Every time you consume protein, your body expends energy to break it down, a phenomenon known as the thermic effect of food. This metabolic boost, coupled with the fat-burning nature of ketosis, creates a powerful combination for weight loss and muscle maintenance.

Take the story of John, a 45-year-old office worker who had tried numerous diets to manage his weight. Despite sticking to calorie-restricted plans, he found himself constantly hungry, fatigued, and frustrated by his lack of progress. After adopting the carnivore diet, John not only lost 20 pounds, but also noticed that his strength in the gym increased. His experience mirrors that of many who turn to the carnivore diet not just for weight loss, but for sustainable and long-term body composition improvements.

But it's not just the average person who benefits from the metabolic shifts of the carnivore diet. Elite athletes have also turned to this way of eating to support their performance goals. The body's ability to efficiently tap into fat stores for fuel leads to better endurance and a leaner physique, without the need for constant carbohydrate replenishment. This metabolic flexibility is one of the reasons so many find the carnivore diet to be a sustainable long-term approach.

Energy Levels and Endurance

One of the unexpected benefits reported by those who adopt the carnivore diet is the surge in energy levels. This is often a pleasant surprise for individuals accustomed to the peaks and valleys associated with carb-heavy diets. The constant need for snacks or meals to stave off fatigue becomes a thing of the past as the body transitions to a fat-burning state.

When carbohydrates are a primary fuel source, energy fluctuations are common. Blood sugar levels rise and fall rapidly, leaving individuals feeling tired or sluggish between meals. On the carnivore diet, however, the body's reliance on fat for fuel leads to more stable energy levels. Fat is a more efficient and long-lasting source of energy, allowing for sustained performance throughout the day.

This shift in energy regulation is particularly beneficial for those engaged in physical activities or demanding jobs. Athletes, in particular, often find that their endurance improves, as the body becomes adept at tapping into fat stores rather than relying on the limited supply of glycogen stored in the muscles. The benefits extend beyond athletic performance, too—many people report that they no longer experience the mid-afternoon crash that was once a regular part of their day.

Sarah, a busy mother of three and a part-time marathon runner, was initially skeptical about switching to a carnivore diet. She feared that without carbohydrates, she wouldn't have the energy to keep up with her kids or train for her races. But after a few weeks of adjusting, Sarah found herself waking up with more energy than she'd had in years. Not only did she complete her marathon training without issue, but she also set a personal record on race day. Stories like Sarah's underscore the power of the carnivore diet to support both everyday energy needs and athletic performance.

Enhanced Digestive Health

Perhaps one of the most surprising benefits of the carnivore diet is the impact it has on digestive health. Conventional wisdom suggests that fiber is essential for digestion, yet many carnivore dieters report improvements in their digestive systems after removing plant-based foods entirely.

While the idea of eliminating fiber may sound counterintuitive, there is growing evidence that certain individuals may benefit from reducing or eliminating fiber, particularly those with conditions like irritable bowel syndrome (IBS), Crohn's disease, or other digestive disorders. The carnivore diet's focus on easily digestible proteins and fats allows the gut to heal and reset. For many, this translates to fewer issues with bloating, gas, and indigestion.

Meat and animal-based foods are highly bioavailable, meaning they are easily absorbed and utilized by the body. Unlike plant foods, which can contain anti-nutrients like lectins and phytates that interfere with digestion and nutrient absorption, animal products are gentle on the gut and provide a steady stream of nutrients. For those who have struggled with digestive discomfort, the simplicity of the carnivore diet can offer relief that other diets have failed to provide.

David, a lifelong sufferer of IBS, had tried every dietary approach recommended by his doctors—low FODMAP, gluten-free, high-fiber—but nothing seemed to alleviate his symptoms. Desperate for a solution, he turned to the carnivore diet. Within weeks, his bloating and stomach cramps had disappeared, and his bathroom habits became regular for the first time in years. While the carnivore diet may not be a one-size-fits-all solution, it has certainly provided life-changing relief for many individuals with digestive issues.

Mental and Cognitive Benefits

While the physical benefits of the carnivore diet are impressive, its impact on mental and cognitive function is equally transformative. Many who adopt this way of eating report sharper focus, better mental clarity, and even improvements in their sleep patterns.

Mental Clarity and Focus

One of the first cognitive benefits many carnivore dieters notice is a profound improvement in mental clarity and focus. Carbohydrates, especially refined sugars and starches, are notorious for causing brain fog and cognitive sluggishness. By eliminating carbs and relying on fat as the primary energy source, the brain receives a more consistent and efficient supply of fuel.

The brain is an energy-intensive organ, consuming roughly 20% of the body's energy. While glucose is often touted as the brain's preferred fuel source, ketones—produced when the body burns fat for fuel—are a more efficient and stable energy source. When the brain runs on ketones, mental clarity and focus are often noticeably improved.

Consider Emily, a high-powered executive who struggled with concentration and productivity in the late afternoons. After switching to the carnivore diet, she found that her mental acuity remained sharp throughout the day. Her work performance improved, and she no longer needed to rely on coffee or energy drinks to stay alert during meetings. The carnivore diet's impact on her cognitive function was one of the most surprising benefits she experienced, and it's one that many others share.

Reduced Brain Fog

In addition to improving focus, the carnivore diet often leads to a reduction in brain fog—a term used to describe feelings of mental cloudiness, forgetfulness, and difficulty concentrating. Brain fog can be caused by a variety of factors, including blood sugar fluctuations, inflammation, and even food sensitivities. By removing plant-based foods that can trigger these issues, many carnivore dieters report that their minds feel clearer and more focused.

Scientific evidence supports the idea that reducing carbohydrates can improve cognitive function. A study published in the Journal of Alzheimer's Disease found that ketogenic diets, which are similar in many ways to the carnivore diet, improved cognitive function in adults with mild cognitive impairment. The study suggests that the brain's use of ketones for energy may help protect against age-related cognitive decline.

The elimination of potential food allergens and inflammatory compounds found in plant foods may also contribute to clearer thinking. Many carnivore dieters who previously struggled with autoimmune conditions or food sensitivities find that their brain fog lifts after making the switch, allowing them to think more clearly and process information more effectively.

Improving Sleep Quality

The carnivore diet not only supports better mental clarity during the day but also has a profound impact on sleep quality. For many, sleep becomes deeper and more restorative after transitioning to this way of eating. While the exact mechanisms behind this improvement are still being studied, several factors likely contribute to better sleep on the carnivore diet.

One potential reason for improved sleep is the regulation of blood sugar levels. On a carbohydrate-heavy diet, blood sugar spikes and crashes can disrupt sleep, leading to restless nights and frequent wake-ups. The carnivore diet's emphasis on fat and protein helps stabilize blood sugar, preventing these disruptions and promoting more restful sleep.

Another factor is the reduction of inflammation. Chronic inflammation is linked to poor sleep quality, and by eliminating inflammatory foods, many carnivore dieters experience a decrease in inflammation-related symptoms, such as joint pain and headaches, that can interfere with sleep. The combination of stable blood sugar, reduced inflammation, and the calming effects of ketones on the brain and body creates the ideal environment for deep, restorative sleep.

For those who have long struggled with insomnia or restless nights, the improvement in sleep quality can be life-changing. Take the example of Michael, a 52-year-old night-shift worker who had battled insomnia for years. After switching to the carnivore diet, he found himself falling asleep faster and waking up feeling refreshed. The diet's impact on his sleep allowed him to handle the demands of his night-shift job without the constant fatigue that had plagued him for years.

The sleep benefits of the carnivore diet extend beyond just feeling well-rested. Quality sleep is foundational for overall health—affecting everything from immune function to mood. When the body is well-rested, it can repair itself more effectively, leading to better physical and mental performance during waking hours. For many, the carnivore diet's positive influence on sleep is one of the most unexpected, yet rewarding, benefits.

Emotional and Psychological Well-being

Beyond the physical and cognitive advantages, the carnivore diet has also been linked to improved emotional and psychological well-being. The connection between diet and mental health is becoming increasingly recognized, and for many, the carnivore diet serves as a tool for not just physical health but also emotional resilience.

Regulating Mood and Anxiety

The carnivore diet has shown promise in helping to regulate mood and reduce anxiety. While traditional advice often focuses on a balanced diet including plant-based foods, research and anecdotal evidence suggest that removing potential triggers like sugar, processed foods, and even certain vegetables can have a calming effect on the mind.

The elimination of carbohydrates and sugars, in particular, plays a key role in this mood stabilization. High-carb, high-sugar diets are notorious for causing erratic blood sugar levels, which can lead to mood swings, irritability, and anxiety. By eliminating these foods and focusing on nutrient-dense animal products, blood sugar remains stable, contributing to more even moods.

Additionally, there is evidence that diets high in healthy fats—like those emphasized in the carnivore diet—support brain health by promoting the production of neurotransmitters such as serotonin and dopamine, which are crucial for mood regulation. A study published in Neuropsychobiology (a peer review scientific journal) found that a diet rich in omega-3 fatty acids (common in fatty fish and grass-fed meats) was associated with reduced symptoms of anxiety and depression. This is why so many carnivore dieters report feeling emotionally balanced and less prone to anxiety after making the dietary shift.

Stress Resilience and Coping Mechanisms

The carnivore diet doesn't just help with mood stabilization—it also appears to enhance resilience to stress. Stress is an inevitable part of life, and how we respond to it can be deeply influenced by our diet. Nutrient deficiencies, inflammation, and fluctuating blood sugar levels can all make it harder for the body to cope with stress. By providing the body with a steady stream of high-quality nutrients, the carnivore diet creates a foundation for emotional resilience.

The diet's impact on inflammation may also play a role in stress resilience. Chronic inflammation has been linked to increased stress reactivity, making it harder for individuals to cope with everyday challenges. By reducing inflammation through the elimination of plant-based irritants and processed foods, the carnivore diet may help buffer the body's response to stress.

For example, Laura, a 38-year-old teacher, had always struggled with stress management. The demands of her job, combined with poor dietary choices, often left her feeling overwhelmed. After adopting the carnivore diet, she found that her capacity to handle stress improved. She was able to remain calm during difficult situations and felt more in control of her emotions. This newfound resilience allowed her to approach both personal and professional challenges with a clearer, more composed mindset.

Boosting Self-Confidence Through Diet

One of the most profound emotional benefits of the carnivore diet is its ability to boost self-confidence. When people feel better physically, mentally, and emotionally, it has a ripple effect on how they view themselves. Weight loss, improved energy levels, enhanced cognitive function, and stable moods can all contribute to a greater sense of self-worth and confidence.

For many, the diet serves as a means of reclaiming control over their health and well-being. The simplicity of the carnivore diet—focusing on nourishing, animal-based foods—gives individuals a sense of empowerment in their choices. Without the constant pressure of counting calories, obsessing over portion sizes, or dealing with cravings, people are able to reconnect with their bodies and trust in their hunger signals.

Take Mark, a 30-year-old former athlete who had gained weight and lost confidence after years of struggling with his diet. The carnivore diet gave him a clear path forward. Within months, he regained his athletic physique and, more importantly, his sense of self-confidence. The physical changes were certainly a factor, but the emotional and psychological benefits were what truly transformed his life. For Mark, the diet wasn't just about eating differently—it was about rediscovering his best self.

Moreover, the self-confidence boost goes beyond personal achievements. The carnivore diet often attracts a community of like-minded individuals who share their experiences and support each other. Being part of a community that understands the challenges and victories of such a unique diet fosters a sense of belonging and camaraderie. This community support can further enhance self-confidence and emotional well-being, creating a positive feedback loop that continues to reinforce the benefits of the diet.

In conclusion, the carnivore diet offers far-reaching benefits that extend well beyond weight loss or improved physical health. From better cognitive function and sleep quality to enhanced emotional resilience and self-confidence, this diet has the potential to transform lives in ways that are both profound and lasting. For those willing to commit to this way of eating, the rewards can be nothing short of life-changing.

CHAPTER 3

Nutritional Myths & Misconceptions

The realm of nutrition is one fraught with controversy, confusion, and misinformation. From conflicting studies to ever-changing dietary guidelines, it's no wonder that many of us are left wondering what's truly good for our health. In the age of processed foods, dietary trends, and the loud voices of "experts," it becomes essential to sift through the noise to uncover the truth. One diet that sits at the heart of modern debate is the carnivore diet—an all-meat regimen that defies nearly every conventional rule of nutrition. With its rise to popularity, the carnivore diet has brought longstanding nutritional myths and misconceptions to the forefront, forcing us to rethink everything from cholesterol to fiber to ethical eating.

This chapter aims to address some of the most pervasive myths in modern nutrition, focusing on key areas of contention and shedding light on the truths that often get lost in mainstream discourse.

Cholesterol and Heart Health

When people first hear about the carnivore diet, one of the first concerns they raise is cholesterol. For decades, we've been told that cholesterol is the primary driver of heart disease, and that eating a diet rich in animal fats will clog our arteries and doom us to an early death. But is this fear justified?

The Cholesterol Debate

The history of cholesterol's vilification dates back to the mid-20th century, when the "lipid hypothesis" gained prominence. This theory, popularized by Ancel Keys, suggested that dietary fat and cholesterol were the main culprits behind rising heart disease rates. Soon after, low-fat diets became the cornerstone of heart health advice, and cholesterol was demonized as a major factor in cardiovascular disease. Yet, over the years, research has painted a more complex picture—one that doesn't fit neatly into the "cholesterol equals heart disease" narrative.

Cholesterol is, in fact, a vital stance for human health. It plays a critical role in the production of hormones, the formation of cell membranes, and even the creation of vitamin D. Rather than being a simple villain, cholesterol is an essential component of life. What's more, our liver produces the majority of the cholesterol in our bodies—regardless of how much we eat. So, why have we been told to fear it?

Emerging research suggests that the connection between dietary cholesterol and heart disease is weak at best. A meta-analysis published in *The American Journal of Clinical Nutrition* in 2015 found no significant link between dietary cholesterol intake and coronary heart disease. What we are beginning to understand is that it's not cholesterol itself, but the context in which it exists within the body that matters.

It's crucial to consider factors such as inflammation, insulin resistance, and oxidative stress, which are more likely to contribute to heart disease than cholesterol alone. Many who switch to a carnivore diet experience reductions in markers of inflammation, improved blood sugar regulation, and better overall metabolic health—factors that contribute to a lower risk of cardiovascular disease.

LDL, HDL, and Triglycerides Explained

When discussing cholesterol, it's important to dive into the different types: LDL (low-density lipoprotein), HDL (high-density lipoprotein), and triglycerides. While cholesterol has long been treated as a monolithic entity, these markers tell us much more about heart health than a total cholesterol number ever could.

LDL is often referred to as "bad" cholesterol, but this is a gross oversimplification. There are different types of LDL, some more harmful than others. Small, dense LDL particles are more likely to contribute to plaque formation in the arteries, while large, fluffy LDL particles are far less problematic. Many people on low-carb or carnivore diets see a rise in their LDL levels, but this often comes alongside an increase in particle size, making the LDL less likely to cause harm.

HDL, on the other hand, is often called "good" cholesterol because it helps transport cholesterol away from the arteries and back to the liver for disposal. On a carnivore diet, many people experience a rise in HDL levels, a sign that their body is efficiently managing cholesterol.

Then there are triglycerides, which are fats carried in the blood. Elevated triglyceride levels are a risk factor for heart disease, and they're often tied to diets high in refined carbohydrates and sugars. On a carnivore diet, triglyceride levels tend to drop significantly as the body shifts to burning fat for fuel instead of carbs. This reduction in triglycerides is one of the most consistent and positive changes people see when switching to a meat-based diet.

Real Heart Health Markers

So, if cholesterol isn't the smoking gun when it comes to heart disease, what should we be looking at? The truth is, heart health is influenced by a wide range of factors, many of which have little to do with the number on a cholesterol panel.

One of the most reliable markers of heart disease risk is inflammation. Elevated levels of C-reactive protein (CRP), a marker of inflammation, have been strongly linked to an increased risk of heart attacks and strokes. The carnivore diet, with its emphasis on whole, unprocessed foods and the elimination of inflammatory plant compounds, often leads to reductions in CRP levels.

Another key marker is insulin sensitivity. Insulin resistance, characterized by chronically elevated blood sugar and insulin levels, is a major driver of heart disease, obesity, and type 2 diabetes. By eliminating carbohydrates, the carnivore diet helps improve insulin sensitivity, allowing the body to manage blood sugar levels more effectively.

Ultimately, when assessing heart disease risk, it's critical to look beyond cholesterol and consider the broader context of metabolic health. A diet rich in nutrient-dense animal products, free from processed foods and inflammatory oils, can offer significant heart health benefits that are often overlooked in the traditional conversation around cholesterol.

Fiber and Gut Health

For years, fiber has been hailed as an essential component of a healthy diet, particularly for its role in digestive health. Yet, the carnivore diet challenges this notion by eliminating fiber entirely. How can a diet devoid of plant-based fiber support gut health, and what role does fiber actually play in our digestive system?

The Role of Fiber—Necessary or Overrated?
The common belief is that fiber is necessary for maintaining regular bowel movements, feeding the microbiome, and preventing digestive disorders such as constipation and colon cancer. However, the reality is not so black and white. While fiber can have benefits for some individuals, it's not essential for everyone, and in certain cases, it may even exacerbate digestive issues.

Fiber works by adding bulk to stool, making it easier to pass through the digestive tract. However, many carnivore dieters report that after an initial adjustment period, they experience regular and healthy bowel movements without fiber. How is this possible? The answer lies in the way our bodies digest and absorb different types of foods.

Animal products are highly bioavailable, meaning they are easily broken down and absorbed by the body, leaving little waste. As a result, those on a carnivore diet tend to produce smaller, less frequent stools because the food they eat is being efficiently utilized by the body. The need for fiber to bulk up the stool becomes less relevant when the digestive system isn't dealing with the indigestible components of plant foods.

Moreover, studies have shown that for some individuals, particularly those with irritable bowel syndrome (IBS) or other gut disorders, reducing or eliminating fiber can actually improve symptoms. A study published in The World *Journal of Gastroenterology* found that a low-fiber diet reduced symptoms of constipation in individuals with IBS. This suggests that the blanket recommendation to increase fiber intake may not be suitable for everyone, particularly those with sensitive digestive systems.

How the Gut Adapts to a Carnivore Diet

The transition to a carnivore diet can be challenging for the digestive system, particularly in the early stages. As the body adapts to processing only animal-based foods, some people may experience digestive discomfort, including constipation or diarrhea. However, these issues are usually temporary as the gut microbiome adjusts to the new diet.

One reason for these short-term digestive changes is the shift in the types of bacteria present in the gut. The gut microbiome—the collection of trillions of bacteria living in our digestive system—plays a critical role in how we process food. On a diet rich in plant-based fiber, certain types of bacteria thrive on fermenting that fiber into short-chain fatty acids. When fiber is removed from the diet, the composition of the microbiome shifts, favoring bacteria that specialize in breaking down animal proteins and fats.

This microbial shift can take time, and some people may experience digestive issues during the transition period. However, once the gut microbiome adapts to the carnivore diet, many individuals report improved digestion, with fewer issues such as bloating, gas, and discomfort.

Microbiome Health Without Plants

One of the most common concerns about the carnivore diet is its impact on the microbiome. We've been told for years that a diverse microbiome, supported by a variety of plant-based foods, is essential for good health. So, how can someone maintain a healthy gut without plants?

While it's true that fiber can feed certain beneficial bacteria, it's not the only way to support a healthy microbiome. The carnivore diet, by providing the body with easily digestible and nutrient-dense foods, creates an environment where gut bacteria can thrive without the need for fiber.

Moreover, recent research has shown that the composition of the microbiome can vary widely between individuals, and there is no one-size-fits-all approach to gut health. A study published in Nature found that gut microbiomes are highly individualized, and what works for one person may not work for another. Some people may thrive on a high-fiber diet, while others may do better with a diet that minimizes or eliminates fiber.

In fact, many carnivore dieters report improvements in gut health after making the switch. This includes reduced bloating, fewer digestive discomforts, and improved regularity—despite the absence of fiber. So, while the conventional wisdom might insist that fiber is indispensable for a healthy gut, real-life experiences on the carnivore diet suggest otherwise. What we're beginning to understand is that the human digestive system is highly adaptable. When provided with the right nutrients, it can thrive even on a diet that breaks all the so-called rules of traditional nutrition.

Additionally, some studies challenge the long-standing notion that a highly diverse microbiome is always better. A study from Cell Host & Microbe indicated that the types of microbes present in the gut, rather than sheer diversity, are what matter most. On the carnivore diet, the gut microbiome may become less diverse, but this isn't inherently a negative outcome. The bacteria that remain are highly efficient at breaking down and absorbing animal nutrients, which is ultimately more relevant to health than simply having a high number of bacterial species.

While the carnivore diet may shift the composition of the gut microbiome, it appears to do so in a way that supports overall digestive health, at least for many individuals. What we're learning is that the relationship between diet, gut bacteria, and health is far more complex than we once believed—and that a lack of fiber does not automatically equate to poor gut health.

Sustainability and Ethical Considerations

One of the major criticisms leveled against the carnivore diet is its perceived impact on the environment and ethical concerns surrounding animal welfare. Can a diet centered on meat be sustainable for the planet? Is it possible to follow a carnivore diet ethically? These are questions that demand careful thought, as they tap into deeply held beliefs about food, health, and the future of the planet.

Is a Meat-Only Diet Environmentally Friendly?

The idea that meat consumption is bad for the environment has become almost gospel in modern discourse. We frequently hear about the carbon footprint of livestock, the resources required to raise animals for food, and the toll that animal agriculture takes on the planet's ecosystems. Yet, the reality is more nuanced.

It's true that factory farming—particularly of grain-fed animals—can have significant environmental impacts. Large-scale industrial farms contribute to greenhouse gas emissions, water pollution, and deforestation. But the carnivore diet doesn't necessarily advocate for supporting this kind of agriculture. Instead, many proponents of the diet emphasize the importance of sourcing meat responsibly, from regenerative farming practices that can actually help restore ecosystems rather than destroy them.

Regenerative agriculture is a farming method that prioritizes soil health, biodiversity, and the natural carbon cycle. By raising animals on pasture, in ways that mimic natural ecosystems, regenerative farming has the potential to sequester more carbon in the soil than it releases, making it a net-positive for the environment. In fact, some studies suggest that properly managed grazing livestock can improve soil quality, enhance water retention, and even reduce the need for synthetic fertilizers, which are a major contributor to greenhouse gas emissions.

For instance, White Oak Pastures, a farm in Georgia, conducted a life-cycle analysis showing that their regenerative farming practices sequestered more carbon than was emitted, making their beef a net carbon sink. This challenges the prevailing narrative that all meat production is environmentally harmful.

Moreover, proponents of the carnivore diet argue that plant-based agriculture is not without its own environmental costs. Large-scale monocropping, which is necessary to produce the vast amounts of grains and vegetables demanded by a plant-based diet, leads to soil depletion, loss of biodiversity, and the use of harmful pesticides and fertilizers. In many ways, plant agriculture can be just as damaging to the environment as poorly managed animal farming.

Thus, when practiced responsibly, a carnivore diet that emphasizes regenerative raised meat can be both sustainable and environmentally friendly. The key is not to view all meat production through the same lens, but rather to focus on the methods used to raise animals.

Humane Sourcing and Ethical Eating

For those concerned about the ethics of eating animals, the carnivore diet raises important questions. Is it possible to eat meat in a way that aligns with ethical values? The answer lies in the way animals are raised, treated, and slaughtered.

Humane sourcing is a cornerstone of ethical eating for carnivore dieters who care about animal welfare. Many who follow the diet advocate for purchasing meat from farms that prioritize animal welfare, ensuring that animals live in natural, healthy environments and are treated with respect throughout their lives. This often means seeking out grass-fed, pasture-raised, and humanely slaughtered meats, where the animals are allowed to graze freely and are not subjected to the cruel conditions of factory farms.

One of the key tenets of ethical meat consumption is the idea that animals should be raised in ways that allow them to express their natural behaviors—such as grazing, rooting, and foraging. When animals are raised on pasture, they can live more in line with their natural instincts, resulting in healthier animals and, arguably, more ethical meat. Many small farms that focus on regenerative agriculture also prioritize these humane practices, creating a more ethical food system.

For example, Polyface Farm, run by farmer and activist Joel Salatin, is renowned for its ethical and sustainable farming methods. Animals at Polyface are rotated on pasture, allowing the land to recover naturally and providing the animals with a high quality of life. This type of farming is a far cry from the factory farms that most people associate with meat production.

Ethical meat consumption also involves being mindful of food waste. Those who follow the carnivore diet often emphasize the importance of eating "nose to tail," which means using as much of the animal as possible—organs, bones, and all. This reduces waste and ensures that every part of the animal is utilized, an important consideration for those concerned about the ethics of meat consumption.

Addressing Ethical Concerns for Vegans and Vegetarians

Perhaps the most contentious aspect of the carnivore diet is its fundamental opposition to veganism and vegetarianism, which are often grounded in ethical concerns about animal rights. How can one reconcile the practice of eating animals with the deeply held belief that all life is sacred?

While it's impossible to resolve this philosophical divide entirely, it's important to engage in a balanced discussion about the ethical trade-offs inherent in all diets. Vegans and vegetarians often argue that their diets cause less harm to animals, but this isn't always the case. Plant agriculture, particularly when practiced on a large scale, can result in the destruction of habitats and the deaths of countless small animals, insects, and birds. Pesticides and industrial farming practices can also have devastating effects on ecosystems and wildlife populations.

In contrast, proponents of the carnivore diet argue that by consuming animals raised on regenerative farms, they are supporting ecosystems rather than depleting them. They contend that animals play an essential role in the natural cycle of life and death, and that by eating animals raised in harmony with the land, they are participating in a more ethical and sustainable food system.

Ultimately, the question of ethics in food is a deeply personal one, and there is no one-size-fits-all answer. What's important is that individuals make informed choices about where their food comes from and how it impacts the world around them. For some, this may mean embracing a plant-based diet; for others, it may mean choosing responsibly sourced animal products.

As we examine the nutritional myths and misconceptions surrounding the carnivore diet, it becomes clear that many of the fears and concerns we've been taught to hold about animal products are rooted in outdated or incomplete science. From cholesterol to fiber to sustainability, the carnivore diet challenges conventional wisdom in profound ways—forcing us to question long-standing assumptions about what truly constitutes a healthy and ethical way of eating.

What this chapter reveals is that nutrition is far more complex and individualized than mainstream advice often suggests. Whether you're considering a carnivore diet for its potential health benefits or simply exploring new perspectives on food, it's worth taking the time to cut through the noise and seek out the truth for yourself. After all, the real power of any diet lies not in its conformity to popular trends, but in its ability to nourish your body and support your overall well-being.

CHAPTER 4

Customizing the Carnivore Diet

The beauty of the carnivore diet lies not just in its simplicity but also in its adaptability. Though it's often portrayed as an all-or-nothing approach, the truth is that the diet can be tailored to fit a wide variety of needs, lifestyles, and preferences. It can be as strict or flexible as you need it to be, depending on your health goals, your daily routine, and even your social commitments. In this chapter, we'll explore how to customize the carnivore diet to make it work for you—whether you're a busy professional, an athlete, or someone grappling with health challenges. This is not a one-size-fits-all approach but rather a framework you can modify to suit your life.

Variations of the Carnivore Diet

The carnivore diet often evokes the image of someone eating steak three times a day, with no room for flexibility. However, there are many variations within the carnivore framework that allow for personalization. Whether you choose to be strict or more lenient, understanding the range of options can help you make the diet sustainable and enjoyable.

Strict Carnivore vs. Carnivore Adjacent

For those who view the carnivore diet as a strict, no-compromise way of eating, the emphasis is entirely on animal products. In this strict interpretation, people consume muscle meats, organ meats, and animal fats while avoiding all plant-based foods. The rationale behind this is to eliminate potential food irritants—like lectins, oxalates, and phytates—commonly found in plants, as well as the carbohydrates that can disrupt metabolic health.

Strict carnivores swear by the simplicity of their approach. They eat only meat and find that their energy, mental clarity, and overall well-being flourish under these conditions. There's no room for negotiation or "cheat days," but for those who thrive on this kind of rigidity, it brings tremendous rewards. It also cuts down on food decisions, which simplifies meal planning and grocery shopping, allowing people to focus on the quality of their food rather than variety.

However, not everyone needs to be this strict. Carnivore adjacent diets allow for some flexibility. This could include adding a few low-toxin plants, like leafy greens or certain fruits, into the diet. While this isn't technically carnivore, it can still provide many of the same benefits while making the diet more palatable for some individuals. Carnivore adjacent diets offer a way to enjoy the best of both worlds—the metabolic benefits of a meat-based diet with a little more flexibility for long-term sustainability.

Adding Minimal Plants or Dairy

For many, the introduction of dairy or minimal plants allows for greater variety without compromising health goals. Dairy products like cheese, cream, and butter can be excellent sources of fat and protein, and some people on the carnivore diet find they tolerate dairy just fine. However, the key is to be selective—full-fat, high-quality dairy from grass-fed cows is far preferable to processed, low-fat options.

Minimal plant additions, like avocado or small amounts of non-starchy vegetables, can also be incorporated, especially for those who aren't dealing with autoimmune issues or severe food sensitivities. These additions help diversify meals without overwhelming the body with carbohydrates. It's important to listen to your body and adjust according to how you feel. Some people thrive on strict carnivore, while others need a bit more leeway to maintain balance.

One noteworthy approach is the use of plants seasonally, following the ancestral patterns of eating what's available during certain times of the year. For example, fruits in summer and autumn might be consumed in small amounts to mimic natural, historical eating patterns. This seasonal approach allows some flexibility without losing the essence of the carnivore framework.

The Zero-Carb Approach

For those who are particularly carb-sensitive or dealing with metabolic disorders like diabetes, the zero-carb approach is a variation that focuses on eliminating all forms of carbohydrates, including from plant sources. This strict interpretation of the carnivore diet involves consuming only meat, fish, eggs, and animal fats. Zero-carb enthusiasts report dramatic improvements in blood sugar control, weight loss, and overall metabolic health.

What makes this approach particularly appealing to some is its ability to induce a state of ketosis, where the body shifts from using glucose for energy to burning fat. Ketones, produced during fat metabolism, provide a steady source of energy for both the brain and body. This metabolic shift is not only advantageous for weight loss but also for improving cognitive function and reducing inflammation.

Zero-carb works particularly well for those who struggle with insulin resistance or autoimmune conditions that seem to be exacerbated by even minimal carbohydrate intake. It's a stricter approach but can be incredibly effective for those who need to control blood sugar or reset their metabolic health entirely.

Adjusting for Lifestyle

One of the challenges many face when adopting any diet is figuring out how to make it work within their busy lives. Whether you're juggling a demanding career, family responsibilities, or a packed workout schedule, it's essential to adapt the carnivore diet to fit your unique lifestyle. The good news is that with a little planning and preparation, it's entirely possible to thrive on the carnivore diet, no matter your circumstances.

The Busy Professional's Plan

For busy professionals who don't have time to cook elaborate meals, the carnivore diet offers a refreshing level of simplicity. Protein-dense, nutrient-packed meals can be made quickly, and with a little preparation, you can ensure that you stay on track even when your schedule is hectic.

One of the best strategies for those with busy schedules is batch cooking. Preparing large quantities of meat on the weekends or during free time allows you to have pre-cooked meals ready to go throughout the week. Whether it's steak, ground beef, or chicken thighs, having ready-to-eat proteins on hand saves time and keeps you from making poor food choices in moments of hunger.

In addition to batch cooking, consider investing in tools like an Instant Pot or air fryer to streamline meal preparation. These appliances can cut down on cooking time and make it easier to prepare meats to your liking with minimal effort. Protein shakes or collagen-rich bone broths are also quick options for busy mornings or on-the-go lunches, ensuring that you stay fueled without resorting to processed or fast food.

Fitness Enthusiast's Carnivore

For those who are heavily into fitness, particularly strength training or endurance sports, the carnivore diet can provide the high-quality protein and fats necessary for muscle repair and energy. One of the main benefits of a meat-based diet is its ability to support lean muscle mass while simultaneously promoting fat loss—a key concern for many athletes.

Athletes on the carnivore diet often report faster recovery times and improved endurance, thanks to the steady energy provided by fats and the anti-inflammatory properties of animal-based nutrients. Protein from animal sources is particularly beneficial for muscle synthesis, and the absence of carbohydrates reduces the risk of bloating, water retention, or inflammation that often accompanies high-carb diets.

To optimize athletic performance on the carnivore diet, it's important to prioritize nutrient-dense foods like organ meats, bone marrow, and fatty cuts of meat. These provide essential vitamins and minerals, including iron, zinc, and B vitamins, that are critical for optimal performance and recovery. Incorporating organ meats such as liver, which is rich in iron and vitamin A, can significantly boost your energy levels and aid in muscle recovery. Athletes who follow the carnivore diet often find that the absence of carbohydrates leads to more stable energy levels, reducing the risk of the energy crashes that can occur with a high-carb diet.

Hydration is also key for fitness enthusiasts. Since the carnivore diet naturally lowers insulin levels, the body excretes more sodium, so replenishing electrolytes—particularly sodium, potassium, and magnesium—is essential. Adding a pinch of high-quality salt to your water or consuming electrolyte supplements can help maintain your energy levels and prevent cramping during intense workouts.

Family-Friendly Carnivore Meals

Adopting a carnivore diet doesn't mean your family has to as well, but it is possible to create meals that can please both you and your loved ones. The key is to focus on simplicity while ensuring that the meals are delicious and satisfying. Start by making the core of the meal carnivore-friendly—for example, grilling steaks, roasting chicken, or slow-cooking pork shoulder—then add sides for the rest of the family if they aren't strictly following the diet.

For families, versatility is crucial. Ground beef is a carnivore staple that can be used to make a variety of family-friendly dishes, from burgers to meatballs. By preparing the protein in bulk, you can use it in different ways throughout the week. You could have burgers one night, taco bowls (with minimal plant additions) the next, and then a meat-based lasagna using layers of ground beef and cheese instead of noodles.

One advantage of the carnivore diet is that it encourages nutrient-dense meals that can benefit the whole family. Even if your children or spouse aren't following the diet strictly, they will still enjoy the benefits of eating real, whole foods with minimal processing. Incorporating fun, creative recipes—like bacon-wrapped meatballs or steak fajitas—makes it easier to get your family on board, even if they include some carbohydrates on the side.

Dietary Challenges and Adjustments

Any dietary shift comes with its challenges, and the carnivore diet is no exception. From sugar cravings to social events, there are practical obstacles you'll need to overcome to stay on track. By addressing these challenges head-on, you can better prepare yourself for the road ahead and learn how to make the diet sustainable for the long term.

Overcoming Sugar Cravings

One of the toughest hurdles for many transitioning to the carnivore diet is overcoming sugar cravings. Our modern diets are filled with sugar and processed carbohydrates, so it's natural to crave these foods during the first few weeks of the diet. The key to overcoming these cravings is to increase your fat intake. Fats are satiating and provide long-lasting energy, which helps curb the desire for sugary foods.

Many people report that within a few weeks of going carnivore, their sugar cravings dramatically decrease. This happens as the body adjusts to using fat for energy instead of glucose. During this adjustment period, it's important to stay hydrated and keep electrolytes balanced, as dehydration can sometimes masquerade as a craving for sugar.

In moments of intense craving, focusing on nutrient-dense, high-fat options like beef tallow, butter, or fatty cuts of meat can help. Some find that consuming small amounts of cheese or cream also helps bridge the gap as the body adapts. If the cravings persist, you can also try incorporating more variety into your meals, like eating different cuts of meat or adding eggs and organ meats for additional texture and flavor.

Dealing with Social Situations

Social events, dining out, and gatherings can be tricky on the carnivore diet, but they are not impossible to navigate. The key is to plan ahead. If you're attending a dinner party or family event, consider bringing a carnivore-friendly dish to share, such as a platter of grilled meats or a hearty roast. This not only ensures that you'll have something to eat but also introduces others to the possibilities of delicious, meat-based meals.

When dining out, most restaurants are willing to accommodate dietary requests. Opt for meat-based dishes like steak, burgers (without the bun), or grilled fish, and ask for substitutions where necessary. You can usually replace sides like potatoes or bread with extra meat or eggs. Avoid sauces or dressings that may contain sugar or processed oils, and don't hesitate to request olive oil or butter as a healthier alternative.

If you're at a social gathering where there are few carnivore-friendly options, focus on eating before you go. This way, you won't feel the need to compromise your diet when faced with less-than-ideal food choices. A small snack of fatty meat or a couple of eggs before you leave home can keep hunger at bay, allowing you to enjoy the event without stress.

Tailoring the Diet for Specific Health Conditions
The carnivore diet can be particularly beneficial for those dealing with specific health conditions, such as autoimmune diseases, metabolic disorders, and digestive issues. However, these individuals may need to make certain adjustments to ensure the diet works for them in the long term.

For those with autoimmune conditions, the strict carnivore approach can help eliminate common food triggers like gluten, lectins, and other plant-based irritants. However, it's important to ensure that your diet is rich in essential nutrients. Organ meats like liver, heart, and kidney provide a concentrated source of vitamins and minerals that can be especially beneficial for those with compromised immune systems.

Individuals with metabolic disorders, such as diabetes or insulin resistance, often see dramatic improvements on the carnivore diet, as it eliminates the blood sugar spikes and crashes associated with carbohydrate consumption. However, they may need to monitor their blood sugar levels more closely during the transition period. It's also important for these individuals to focus on nutrient-dense sources of protein and fat to stabilize blood sugar and support metabolic health.

For those dealing with digestive issues like irritable bowel syndrome (IBS) or Crohn's disease, the carnivore diet can offer relief by eliminating fiber and plant-based irritants. However, transitioning to an all-meat diet can require some adjustment. In the short term, some individuals may experience digestive discomfort as their bodies adapt to the increased intake of animal products. Drinking bone broth, consuming fermented foods, and slowly introducing different cuts of meat can ease the transition and support gut healing.

In conclusion, the carnivore diet's simplicity is one of its greatest strengths, but its adaptability is what makes it truly sustainable. Whether you're a busy professional, a dedicated athlete, or someone dealing with specific health challenges, the diet can be customized to fit your unique needs and goals. By understanding the various approaches, staying flexible, and addressing challenges proactively, you can create a carnivore lifestyle that enhances your well-being while remaining practical for your everyday life.

CHAPTER 5

Carnivore Diet & Longevity

As the quest for longevity has become the cornerstone of modern wellness, diets promising youth, vitality, and disease prevention have garnered enormous attention. From intermittent fasting to plant-based regimes, many have proclaimed their superiority in the race for prolonged life. However, emerging science and anecdotal evidence suggest that the carnivore diet might have a unique place in this discussion. At its core, the carnivore diet—a regimen that prioritizes animal-based nutrition—offers not only fundamental nourishment but also remarkable potential in extending both lifespan and healthspan. In this chapter, we delve into how the carnivore diet can directly impact longevity by preserving physical strength, warding off chronic disease, and safeguarding mental clarity well into old age.

Anti-Aging Benefits

In the discussion of aging, it's common to focus on superficial aspects like wrinkles or gray hair. But true longevity isn't just about living longer—it's about living well, maintaining muscle mass, strong bones, and a youthful radiance that belies your years. The carnivore diet plays a critical role in supporting these aspects of physical health.

The Role of Protein in Preserving Muscle Mass

Aging is often accompanied by sarcopenia, the gradual loss of muscle mass and strength that begins in our 30s and accelerates with each passing decade. This decline isn't just an aesthetic issue—it directly affects mobility, balance, and overall quality of life. Research consistently shows that preserving muscle mass is a key factor in healthy aging, and this is where the carnivore diet excels.

Protein, particularly from animal sources, is the building block of muscle tissue. Animal protein is superior to plant protein in terms of amino acid composition and bioavailability, meaning that your body can more efficiently use the protein from meat to build and maintain muscle. According to a study published in *The American Journal of Clinical Nutrition*, individuals who consume adequate amounts of high-quality protein are significantly less likely to experience age-related muscle loss. The carnivore diet, which is inherently high in animal protein, provides the necessary tools to maintain and even build muscle well into your later years.

Athletes and fitness enthusiasts have long known the power of protein in muscle preservation, but its importance extends beyond the gym. As we age, maintaining muscle isn't just about performance—it's about independence. The ability to walk, climb stairs, and lift everyday objects without assistance is tied to having strong, functional muscles. By ensuring that protein remains a core part of your diet, particularly in the form of nutrient-dense animal foods, you are setting yourself up for a more active and independent old age.

Collagen and Skin Health: Why Carnivores May Have a Youthful Glow
Beyond muscle, the skin is one of the most visible markers of aging. Collagen, the most abundant protein in the body, is a structural component of skin, providing it with elasticity, strength, and the ability to recover from wear and tear. As we age, collagen production naturally declines, leading to sagging, wrinkles, and thinning skin. However, consuming a diet rich in collagen—such as that found in animal products like bone broth, skin, and connective tissue—can help combat these visible signs of aging.

The carnivore diet is inherently rich in collagen-boosting foods. Bone broth, a staple for many carnivores, is particularly beneficial. Packed with collagen, gelatin, and essential minerals, it has been celebrated for its ability to support joint health, improve skin elasticity, and even promote better sleep. Anecdotal reports from carnivore diet followers frequently highlight improvements in skin health, with many claiming a clearer complexion and a more youthful appearance.

But it's not just about looking good. Collagen also plays a vital role in wound healing and tissue repair, making it an essential nutrient for aging gracefully. A study in the *Journal of Cosmetic*

Dermatology showed that regular consumption of collagen peptides led to significant improvements in skin hydration and elasticity, demonstrating that what you eat can have a direct impact on how you age.

Bone Health and Longevity: Strong Bones Through Meat and Marrow

Fragile bones are another common concern as we age. Osteoporosis, a condition characterized by weak and brittle bones, affects millions of people worldwide, particularly post-menopausal women. While calcium is often touted as the solution to strong bones, recent research suggests that dietary protein, especially from animal sources, plays an equally important role in bone health.

Animal-based foods are rich in bioavailable calcium, phosphorus, and vitamin D—all of which are critical for maintaining bone density. Meat and bone marrow, in particular, provide a readily absorbable form of calcium that the body can use to strengthen bones. Furthermore, the protein found in meat helps increase the production of collagen, which is essential for the structural integrity of bones.

A study published in *The Journal of Bone and Mineral Research* found that higher protein intake was associated with greater bone density and a lower risk of fractures in older adults. Contrary to the outdated belief that a high-protein diet leaches calcium from the bones, modern research shows that adequate protein intake actually supports bone health, especially when combined with other nutrients like vitamin D and magnesium.

The carnivore diet, which naturally includes foods like fatty cuts of meat, organ meats, and marrow, provides the perfect balance of nutrients to support lifelong bone health, making it a powerful tool in the fight against osteoporosis and fractures.

Preventing Chronic Disease

Chronic diseases such as diabetes, heart disease, and cancer are the leading causes of death worldwide. Many of these conditions are tied to modern dietary patterns—high in processed foods, refined sugars, and unhealthy fats. The carnivore diet, with its emphasis on whole, nutrient-dense animal foods, offers a compelling alternative that may help prevent and even reverse these conditions.

Reversing Insulin Resistance: A Deep Dive Into Metabolic Health

Insulin resistance, a condition in which the body's cells become less responsive to the hormone insulin, is a precursor to type 2 diabetes and is closely linked to obesity, heart disease, and other metabolic disorders. The modern diet, heavy in refined carbohydrates and sugars, is a major driver of insulin resistance. However, the carnivore diet—devoid of carbohydrates—offers a way to reverse this dangerous condition.

By eliminating carbs, the carnivore diet forces the body to rely on fat for fuel, a metabolic state known as ketosis. In ketosis, insulin levels remain low and stable, allowing the body's cells to become more sensitive to insulin over time. This not only helps prevent blood sugar spikes but also reduces inflammation, a key factor in the development of insulin resistance.

A study published in Diabetes Therapy showed that a low-carb, high-fat diet led to significant improvements in insulin sensitivity and blood sugar control in individuals with type 2 diabetes. Many people who adopt the carnivore diet report similar benefits, with some even able to reduce or eliminate their need for diabetes medications.

Heart Disease Prevention: The Real Impact of a Carnivore Diet on Cardiovascular Health

Heart disease has long been the number one killer in many parts of the world, and for decades, dietary fat—particularly saturated fat—has been blamed. However, recent research has called into question the role of saturated fat in heart disease, and many experts now believe that inflammation and insulin resistance, rather than dietary fat, are the true culprits.

The carnivore diet, rich in healthy fats and free from refined carbohydrates, addresses these root causes of heart disease. By reducing inflammation and stabilizing blood sugar levels, the carnivore diet may help lower the risk of heart disease. Furthermore, studies have shown that cholesterol levels—particularly LDL and HDL—are more complex than previously thought. It's now clear that having higher levels of HDL (the so-called "good" cholesterol) is protective, and many people on the carnivore diet report improvements in their cholesterol profiles, with higher HDL levels and a better LDL-to-HDL ratio.

One study published in the *British Journal of Nutrition* found that individuals who consumed a high-protein, low-carb diet had better cardiovascular health markers than those on a low-fat diet. This challenges the traditional notion that fat is the enemy, suggesting instead that a diet rich in animal protein and fat can support heart health.

Cancer and the Carnivore Diet: Examining the Evidence for Anti-Cancer Properties
Cancer is a complex and multifaceted disease, but there is growing interest in how diet may influence its development and progression. While no diet can guarantee cancer prevention, there is evidence to suggest that the carnivore diet, by reducing inflammation and stabilizing blood sugar levels, may help lower cancer risk.

Many cancers are fueled by high insulin levels and chronic inflammation, both of which are driven by the consumption of refined carbohydrates and sugars. The carnivore diet, which eliminates these foods, may help create an environment in the body that is less conducive to cancer growth. Additionally, some studies have shown that ketosis, the metabolic state induced by the carnivore diet, may inhibit the growth of certain types of cancer cells.

A study published in Cell Metabolism found that restricting glucose in the diet inhibited the growth of cancer cells in mice, suggesting that a low-carb, high-fat diet could have anti-cancer effects. While more research is needed in humans, these findings are promising and provide a strong rationale for further exploring the potential benefits of the carnivore diet in cancer prevention.

Cognitive and Neurological Longevity

As we age, cognitive decline becomes a growing concern for many. Alzheimer's disease, dementia, and other neurodegenerative conditions can significantly impact quality of life in later years. However, there is mounting evidence that diet, particularly a low-carb, high-fat diet like the carnivore diet, may help protect brain health and enhance cognitive function well into old age.

Protecting Brain Health as You Age

The brain relies on a steady supply of energy to function optimally, and the carnivore diet provides a consistent source of energy in the form of fat. When the body enters a state of ketosis—burning fat for fuel instead of carbohydrates—ketones become the primary energy source for the brain. Research suggests that ketones are not only a more efficient fuel for the brain, but also have neuroprotective effects.

One of the main threats to brain health as we age is oxidative stress, which damages cells and contributes to cognitive decline. Ketones have been shown to reduce oxidative stress and inflammation in the brain, which may help protect against neurodegenerative conditions like Alzheimer's and Parkinson's disease. A study published in Frontiers in Molecular Neuroscience found that ketones can enhance mitochondrial function and reduce the accumulation of damaging proteins associated with Alzheimer's, offering hope for those at risk of cognitive decline.

Moreover, the carnivore diet's emphasis on nutrient-dense animal foods provides essential nutrients like omega-3 fatty acids, vitamin B12, and choline—all of which are critical for brain health. Omega-3s, in particular, have been linked to improved cognitive function and a reduced risk of dementia. By prioritizing foods rich in these brain-boosting nutrients, the carnivore diet may help preserve mental clarity and sharpness as you age.

Alzheimer's and Diet: The Carnivore Connection to Brain Diseases

Alzheimer's disease is often referred to as "type 3 diabetes" because of its strong connection to insulin resistance and impaired glucose metabolism in the brain. As the brain becomes less efficient at using glucose for energy, cognitive decline accelerates. This is where the carnivore diet, with its ability to induce ketosis and provide an alternative fuel source for the brain, comes into play.

Several studies have shown that a ketogenic diet—similar to the carnivore diet—can improve cognitive function in individuals with Alzheimer's and other forms of dementia. A study published in Neurobiology of Aging found that individuals with mild cognitive impairment who followed a ketogenic diet experienced significant improvements in memory and cognitive performance. These findings suggest that by reducing insulin resistance and providing the brain with ketones for fuel, the carnivore diet may offer protection against Alzheimer's and other neurodegenerative diseases.

Furthermore, animal-based foods are rich in nutrients that support brain health and reduce inflammation, both of which are key factors in preventing Alzheimer's. For example, choline, found in egg yolks and liver, is essential for the production of acetylcholine, a neurotransmitter involved in memory and learning. Vitamin B12, found exclusively in animal products, is also critical for brain function, and deficiencies in B12 have been linked to cognitive decline.

By providing the brain with the nutrients it needs to thrive and protecting it from the damaging effects of insulin resistance, the carnivore diet may offer a powerful defense against Alzheimer's and other brain diseases.

Enhancing Cognitive Function in Later Years: Real-Life Stories of Mental Agility
A growing number of individuals who follow the carnivore diet report not only physical health improvements but also enhanced mental clarity and cognitive function well into their later years. These anecdotal stories are backed by emerging scientific evidence that suggests a meat-based diet can support cognitive health and prevent mental decline.

One such story is that of Dr. Shawn Baker, a leading advocate of the carnivore diet and author of The Carnivore Diet. In his late 50s, Baker has reported increased mental sharpness, improved memory, and sustained focus, all of which he attributes to his meat-based diet. Baker's experience is not unique—many people on the carnivore diet have shared similar stories of improved brain function, sharper focus, and better memory.

These real-life accounts, coupled with the scientific evidence supporting the neuroprotective benefits of ketones and the nutrient density of animal foods, paint a compelling picture of how the carnivore diet can enhance cognitive function in later years. Whether it's maintaining mental agility, preventing brain fog, or simply feeling sharper and more focused, the carnivore diet may hold the key to unlocking lifelong cognitive health.

Conclusion

The carnivore diet, with its emphasis on nutrient-dense animal foods and its ability to induce ketosis, offers a unique approach to longevity and cognitive health. By preserving muscle mass, supporting bone health, and providing the brain with a steady source of ketones, the carnivore diet may help prevent the physical and mental decline that often accompanies aging.

Moreover, the diet's potential to reverse insulin resistance, reduce inflammation, and lower the risk of chronic diseases like heart disease, diabetes, and Alzheimer's makes it a powerful tool for extending both lifespan and healthspan. While more research is needed to fully understand the long-term effects of the carnivore diet, the early evidence is promising, and many individuals are already experiencing the benefits of this meat-based approach to health and longevity.

In a world where the pursuit of youth and vitality often leads to extreme diets and unproven supplements, the carnivore diet offers a natural, nutrient-rich alternative that has stood the test of time. By returning to the ancestral roots of human nutrition and embracing the healing power of animal foods, we can unlock the secrets to a long, healthy, and vibrant life.

CHAPTER 6

The Emotional Journey of the Carnivore Diet

The Carnivore Diet is often discussed in terms of its physical benefits—improved health markers, increased energy levels, and weight loss, to name a few. However, one of the most transformative aspects of this way of eating is the emotional journey that accompanies it. Embracing a meat-only diet is not just about changing what you eat; it's about fundamentally shifting how you relate to food, your body, and even the world around you.

This journey is full of emotional highs and lows, self-discovery, and the eventual building of unshakable confidence. It is a path that stabilizes mood swings, fosters resilience in the face of criticism, and helps you connect with a community of like-minded individuals who can support you every step of the way.

Emotional Benefits

Stabilizing Mood Swings: How Cutting Carbs Reduces Emotional Volatility

For many people, the link between diet and mood is undeniable. While carbohydrates and sugary foods can offer a temporary emotional lift, the crash that follows often leads to irritability, fatigue, and emotional volatility. The carnivore diet, which eliminates processed carbs and sugars, provides a more stable source of energy, which has a profound effect on emotional regulation.

When you cut out the highs and lows caused by fluctuating blood sugar levels, you naturally stabilize your mood. Research has shown that diets high in refined carbohydrates can contribute to mood swings and even depressive symptoms. By eliminating these from your diet, you create a biochemical environment in which your mood remains more balanced throughout the day.

Many carnivores report feeling calmer and more emotionally grounded within just a few weeks of starting the diet. They no longer experience the "hanger" (hunger-fueled anger) or the late-afternoon energy crashes that lead to frustration and irritability. Instead, their emotional state becomes more predictable and consistent, allowing them to navigate life's challenges with a greater sense of ease.

One carnivore diet advocate, Kelly Hogan, shared that after switching to an all-meat diet, she noticed significant improvements in her mood stability. No longer subject to the emotional rollercoaster of sugar highs and lows, she found herself feeling more patient and less reactive in stressful situations. This emotional steadiness, she says, has been one of the most surprising benefits of the carnivore lifestyle.

Food and Happiness Correlation: Emotional Upliftment Through Dietary Choices

It's often said that "you are what you eat," but how often do we stop to consider the emotional impact of our food choices? On the carnivore diet, the simplicity of meals can lead to an unexpected sense of emotional freedom. Instead of obsessing over portion sizes, calorie counting, or meal timing, carnivores focus on eating nutrient-dense foods until they're satisfied.

This simplicity allows for a reconnection with the primal joy of eating—an experience many of us have lost in the world of overly complicated diets and processed foods. The psychological relief of knowing exactly what to eat and when can lead to a deeper sense of happiness and fulfillment. No longer trapped in the cycle of restrictive eating or guilty indulgence, carnivores often report feeling liberated from the emotional baggage that many other diets bring.

Additionally, there is growing research suggesting that animal-based foods can support emotional well-being through the direct impact of nutrients like omega-3 fatty acids, vitamin B12, and zinc. Omega-3s, found in abundance in fatty cuts of meat and fish, are known to play a critical role in brain health and have been linked to reduced symptoms of depression. By nourishing the brain with these essential nutrients, carnivores can experience an uplift in their emotional state that transcends mere mood stabilization.

Building Confidence in Your Choices: Empowerment from Aligning Health with Goals

One of the most powerful emotional shifts that occur on the carnivore diet is the development of confidence. As you begin to see positive changes in your health, energy, and mood, you naturally start to trust your body's signals more and feel more empowered by the choices you're making.

This empowerment is not just about physical transformation but also about gaining confidence in your ability to follow through on your goals. Sticking to the carnivore diet requires discipline and self-awareness, but with each passing day, you build the inner resilience to stay committed. Over time, this leads to a profound sense of pride and self-sufficiency that extends far beyond the plate.

Feeling confident in your dietary choices can also reduce anxiety and second-guessing, especially when confronted with social pressures or outside criticism. Knowing that you are taking control of your health by aligning your eating habits with your personal goals fosters a deep sense of accomplishment and personal power. As many carnivores have discovered, this confidence radiates into other areas of life, enhancing relationships, work, and even creative pursuits.

Coping with Criticism and Skepticism

Dealing with Naysayers and Skeptics: Responding to Critics in Social Settings

It's no secret that the carnivore diet is often met with skepticism, if not outright criticism. Whether from friends, family, or medical professionals, those who choose this lifestyle may encounter questions, concerns, and even judgment. Navigating these social dynamics can be one of the most emotionally challenging aspects of the carnivore journey, but it also provides an opportunity for growth.

The key to handling naysayers is rooted in knowledge and confidence. Understanding the science behind the diet and being able to articulate your reasons for choosing it can disarm critics and open up productive conversations. It's important to remember that many people's skepticism stems from unfamiliarity or misinformation, and your calm, informed responses can often shift their perspective.

When faced with criticism in social settings, it's helpful to take a non-confrontational approach. Instead of feeling defensive or pressured to justify your choices, try framing your response as a personal experience: "This way of eating has worked incredibly well for me, and I feel better than I have in years." By sharing your own success without pushing it on others, you create space for curiosity rather than conflict.

Trusting Your Body's Signals: Learning to Rely on Personal Experience Over External Opinions

One of the most empowering aspects of the carnivore diet is learning to trust your own body's signals. In a world filled with conflicting dietary advice, it's easy to feel confused or overwhelmed by external opinions. However, the simplicity of the carnivore diet allows you to tune in more closely to your body's needs and responses.

As you begin to notice improvements in your health—whether it's increased energy, better digestion, or clearer skin—you develop a deeper trust in your body's ability to guide you. This internal feedback becomes more reliable than any external advice, and over time, you may find yourself less swayed by the opinions of others.

Many carnivores report that this heightened body awareness becomes a powerful tool for navigating life's challenges. Whether it's adjusting your diet to support specific health goals or simply knowing when to rest or push harder in the gym, trusting your body's signals builds a stronger connection to yourself and reinforces your sense of autonomy.

Maintaining Motivation on Tough Days: Strategies for Staying Committed to the Diet

No diet is without its challenges, and the carnivore diet is no exception. There will be days when cravings hit, social situations feel awkward, or the monotony of eating the same foods may start to wear on you. However, it's in these moments that your commitment to the diet—and to yourself—will be tested.

Staying motivated on tough days often comes down to remembering your "why." Why did you start this diet in the first place? What health goals are you working toward? Reconnecting with your reasons for choosing this lifestyle can reignite your motivation and help you push through moments of doubt.

Another powerful strategy is to track your progress. Whether it's keeping a food journal, taking progress photos, or measuring improvements in your health markers, having tangible evidence of your success can be incredibly motivating. It's easy to forget how far you've come when you're in the middle of a tough day, but looking back at your progress can remind you of the incredible changes you've already achieved.

Community and Support

Finding Like-Minded People: Where to Connect with Fellow Carnivores

The emotional journey of the carnivore diet can feel isolating at times, especially if you don't know anyone else following the same path. However, one of the greatest resources available to you is the growing community of carnivores around the world.

Connecting with like-minded individuals who share your dietary approach can provide invaluable emotional support and encouragement. Whether it's through online forums, social media groups, or local meetups, finding your tribe can make all the difference in staying committed to the diet.

Many carnivores find that sharing their experiences with others not only helps them stay motivated but also deepens their sense of belonging. Knowing that you're not alone in your journey can alleviate feelings of isolation and provide a sense of camaraderie that bolsters your emotional well-being.

Online and Local Support Groups: The Role of Social Support in Diet Success

The importance of social support cannot be overstated when it comes to the success of any lifestyle change, and the carnivore diet is no exception. Online support groups, in particular, offer a convenient and accessible way to connect with others who are on the same journey. These groups provide a platform for sharing tips, recipes, and personal stories, as well as offering encouragement during challenging times.

Local support groups, although less common, can also provide a valuable sense of community. Whether it's meeting up for carnivore-friendly meals or attending health-focused events, being around others who understand and support your dietary choices can reinforce your commitment and help you navigate the emotional ups and downs of the journey.

Inspiring Others with Your Journey: Sharing Your Progress and Influencing Change

As you progress on your carnivore journey, something unexpected often happens—you begin to inspire others. Whether it's family members, friends, or even strangers online, people take notice when someone achieves significant health improvements or displays a newfound sense of confidence and vitality. This is where the emotional aspect of the diet comes full circle: not only are you benefiting from the physical and mental changes, but your journey becomes a source of motivation for those around you.

Sharing your progress doesn't have to mean proselytizing or pressuring others to adopt the carnivore diet. Instead, simply sharing your story—your challenges, victories, and how the diet has transformed your life—can plant seeds of curiosity and inspiration in others. Many carnivores have found that by leading by example, they influence people in their circle to make healthier dietary choices, even if those choices don't align perfectly with the carnivore approach.

The ripple effect of your journey extends beyond just food. When people see you taking charge of your health, sticking to your goals, and thriving in ways they didn't think possible, they are more likely to examine their own habits and beliefs. You become a beacon of what's possible, showing others that there's a different, and often better, way to nourish the body and mind.

In many cases, the act of sharing your story also deepens your own sense of commitment to the diet. As you reflect on your progress and communicate it to others, you reinforce your reasons for choosing the carnivore lifestyle and strengthen your resolve to continue. By helping others, you ultimately help yourself.

Final Thoughts on the Emotional Journey of the Carnivore Diet

The emotional journey that accompanies the carnivore diet is as profound and transformative as the physical changes it brings. It's a journey that invites you to reevaluate your relationship with food, build a stronger sense of self-confidence, and connect with a community of like-minded individuals who support your goals. From stabilizing mood swings to coping with criticism, the carnivore diet offers an emotional transformation that many people don't anticipate when they first start.

As you progress on this journey, you'll likely find that the most significant changes are not just on the scale or in your health markers, but in your mindset and emotional well-being. You'll learn to trust your body, build resilience in the face of challenges, and gain a deep sense of satisfaction from aligning your dietary choices with your health goals. Along the way, you'll inspire others and become part of a growing community that's redefining what it means to live a healthy, fulfilled life.

The emotional journey of the carnivore diet is ultimately about empowerment—empowerment to take control of your health, make choices that align with your values, and live a life that is not dictated by the ever-changing tides of conventional dietary advice. It's about finding what works for you, embracing that path fully, and sharing your journey with others who may be seeking the same kind of transformation.

CHAPTER 7

Carnivore Diet Recipes & Meal Plans

Transitioning to the carnivore diet can feel like venturing into a culinary unknown. But once you understand the simplicity and beauty of this way of eating, your kitchen will become a sanctuary for robust flavors, satisfying meals, and optimal nutrition. The carnivore lifestyle is more than just eating meat—it's about embracing the richness of animal-based foods and learning how to transform them into delicious, nourishing meals. In this chapter, we'll explore the essentials you need in your pantry, provide you with structured meal plans to ease into this lifestyle, and introduce a variety of creative recipes that will make your carnivore journey as satisfying as it is sustainable.

Essentials for Your Pantry

Must-Have Ingredients for the Carnivore Kitchen

When embarking on the carnivore diet, the first step is to stock your kitchen with high-quality ingredients that will fuel your body and excite your taste buds. While the simplicity of this diet may seem limiting at first glance, you'll soon discover that with the right ingredients, you can create meals that are both diverse and deeply satisfying. The heart of the carnivore pantry is, of course, meat—but not just any meat. Grass-fed beef, pasture-raised pork, wild-caught fish, and free-range poultry are staples that provide superior nutrition and flavor compared to their factory-farmed counterparts.

In addition to muscle meat, it's essential to include organ meats, which are nutrient powerhouses. Liver, heart, and kidney might sound intimidating, but they are vital for a well-rounded carnivore diet, offering a concentrated source of vitamins, minerals, and healthy fats. Bone marrow, another overlooked gem, provides collagen, which supports skin, joint, and bone health, making it a cornerstone of a diet focused on longevity.

Healthy fats are the other crucial component. Tallow, ghee, and duck fat are excellent for cooking and adding richness to meals. These fats not only add flavor but also provide the energy necessary for those following a ketogenic, low-carb carnivore lifestyle. Lastly, eggs—nature's perfect package—should always have a place in your pantry. Rich in protein, vitamins, and healthy fats, eggs are incredibly versatile and can be used in countless carnivore-friendly dishes.

Preparing Proteins Like a Pro

The carnivore diet hinges on mastering the art of cooking proteins to perfection. Unlike the plant-heavy diets many people are accustomed to, the carnivore way of eating celebrates the richness of animal-based foods, with cooking techniques that enhance their natural flavors and textures. Whether you're searing a ribeye steak or slow-roasting a pork shoulder, there are a few basic principles that will elevate your cooking.

When it comes to beef, searing is key. A hot pan or grill locks in the juices and creates a flavorful crust. Don't shy away from fat—it's what makes the carnivore diet so satisfying. Let that fat render down, basting your meat as it cooks, and you'll have a juicy, melt-in-your-mouth steak every time. For slower-cooked meats, like pork and lamb, the secret lies in low-and-slow cooking. Using a Dutch oven or a slow cooker allows the collagen in the meat to break down, resulting in tender, fall-apart meat that's perfect for family dinners or meal prepping.

Fish and seafood bring variety to the carnivore diet. Grilling or pan-frying wild-caught fish like salmon or cod is quick and easy, while shellfish like shrimp and scallops add a luxurious touch to any meal. For poultry, roasting a whole chicken with its skin on not only keeps it juicy but also gives you the added benefit of crispy skin—one of the delights of carnivore eating.

Quick, Simple Carnivore Snacks

While meals on the carnivore diet are often hearty and filling, having a few quick snack options on hand can make the transition smoother, especially for beginners. One of the simplest and most nutritious snacks is beef jerky. When made from high-quality meat without added sugar or preservatives, jerky provides a convenient, protein-packed option that's easy to take on the go.

Another great snack is pork rinds—crispy, salty, and satisfying. These can be found in most stores or made at home by frying pork skin until puffed and golden. They're perfect for satisfying crunchy cravings without deviating from the carnivore framework.

Hard-boiled eggs are another versatile snack that's quick to prepare and rich in nutrients. They're portable and can be eaten on their own or with a sprinkle of salt for added flavor. And for those looking for something a bit more indulgent, slices of cheese or a handful of cold-smoked salmon can add a touch of luxury to your snack options, without compromising your dietary goals.

Daily Meal Plans

7-Day Beginner Meal Plan

For those new to the carnivore diet, it's essential to keep things simple and manageable in the first week. The following 7-day meal plan is designed to help you transition smoothly, focusing on easy-to-prepare meals that require minimal cooking skills while ensuring you get all the nutrients you need.

On Day 1, start with a breakfast of scrambled eggs cooked in butter, paired with crispy bacon. For lunch, enjoy a grilled chicken breast with a side of bone broth for added collagen. Dinner can be a classic ribeye steak, seared in ghee, and served with a side of beef liver pâté for an extra nutrient boost.

As the week progresses, you'll find a rhythm. Rotate between beef, pork, chicken, and seafood for variety. Try incorporating organ meats gradually, perhaps by blending liver into ground beef for a nutrient-packed burger. By Day 7, you'll feel more comfortable experimenting with different cuts of meat, adding rich flavors through cooking techniques like braising and roasting.

Advanced Meal Plan for Long-Term Success

Once you've adjusted to the carnivore lifestyle, you can begin to explore more diverse meal options that cater to your preferences and nutritional goals. An advanced meal plan introduces more complexity, with meals that require longer cooking times but offer even greater rewards in terms of flavor and texture.

Start your day with a rich carnivore omelet, filled with crumbled sausage, bacon, and a sprinkle of cheese if you tolerate dairy. Lunch might be slow-cooked lamb shanks, which fall off the bone after hours of braising in bone broth. For dinner, consider a roasted duck breast with crispy skin, served alongside a decadent beef marrow bone, the gelatinous marrow acting as a rich, nutritious side.

This plan also encourages the inclusion of more seafood, such as grilled sardines or butter-poached lobster tails. These meals not only offer variety but also ensure you're getting a range of vitamins and minerals that support long-term health on the carnivore diet.

Meals for Special Occasions

Just because you're following a carnivore diet doesn't mean you have to miss out on special occasions. Whether it's a holiday feast or a casual get-together with friends, there are plenty of ways to stay carnivore while enjoying the festivities.

For a celebratory dinner, consider roasting a whole prime rib, served with a side of herb-crusted lamb chops. A rich gravy made from the roasting juices can elevate the meal, and for a special treat, finish with a decadent dessert like a carnivore-friendly custard made from eggs and heavy cream.

If you're attending a social gathering, stick to simple, crowd-pleasing dishes like bacon-wrapped scallops or mini meatballs made from ground beef and pork. These can be served with dipping sauces made from bone broth reductions or rich aioli. By preparing ahead and bringing a dish that aligns with your diet, you'll ensure that you can stay a carnivore without feeling like you're missing out.

Delicious and Creative Carnivore Recipes

Breakfast Options

Starting the day with a carnivore-friendly breakfast doesn't have to be monotonous. While eggs and bacon are a classic, there are other options to keep things exciting. Try a breakfast steak topped with a fried egg, or a rich salmon frittata made with wild-caught fish, eggs, and a touch of cream.

For those in a rush, carnivore smoothies made from raw eggs, cream, and a spoonful of collagen powder can provide a quick, nutrient-dense start to the day. These shakes are creamy, filling, and packed with everything you need to fuel your morning.

Nourishing Lunch and Dinner Ideas

Lunch and dinner on the carnivore diet are the meals where you can really indulge. One favorite is braised short ribs, cooked low and slow until the meat is falling off the bone. Serve with a rich, reduced sauce made from the cooking juices, and you've got a meal that feels both luxurious and comforting.

For a quick lunch, ground beef or bison patties are a great option. Grill them with a slice of cheese on top, and pair them with a few slices of crispy bacon for added flavor. Another dinner favorite is pan-seared duck breast, which delivers a crispy, golden skin and tender, juicy meat—perfect for an elegant yet simple meal.

Indulgent Treats and Drinks

Even on the carnivore diet, there are moments when you might crave something a little indulgent. For a special treat, try making carnivore ice cream using heavy cream, egg yolks, and a touch of vanilla. This rich, creamy dessert satisfies cravings while keeping you firmly within your dietary boundaries.

Carnivore-friendly beverages, such as bone broth lattes, made by blending bone broth with butter or ghee, offer a warm, comforting drink that's both nourishing and delicious. These drinks can be a perfect pick-me-up between meals, providing essential nutrients while keeping you satiated.

CHAPTER 8

Sustaining Long-Term Success

Embracing the carnivore diet is not just about the first few weeks or even the first few months—it is about creating a lifestyle that endures. For those who choose this path, sustaining long-term success requires more than simply eating meat. It calls for a holistic approach that integrates health, motivation, and purpose into daily life. In this chapter, we will explore the strategies and insights necessary to maintain the benefits of the carnivore diet for years to come. We'll delve into measuring long-term health, overcoming plateaus, and ensuring that this way of eating becomes a seamless part of your life.

Measuring Long-Term Health Markers

Tracking Blood Work and Biometrics: What to Watch For

As you continue on the carnivore diet, one of the most important aspects of sustaining long-term success is understanding your health markers. Monitoring blood work and other biometrics is essential not only for tracking progress, but also for making adjustments that enhance well-being. While weight loss, energy levels, and mental clarity are often noticeable within the first few weeks, the deeper, more the changes in health may take longer to emerge—and these changes are best measured through blood tests and biometric tracking.

Regular blood work should be part of your long-term health strategy on the carnivore diet. Important metrics to track include lipid panels, inflammatory markers, insulin sensitivity, and kidney and liver function. Many people on the carnivore diet report improvements in cholesterol levels, with an increase in HDL (the "good" cholesterol) and a reduction in triglycerides, which are both positive signs for cardiovascular health. Contrary to outdated misconceptions, dietary cholesterol does not equate to high cholesterol levels in the blood. Instead, the composition of your diet can lead to improved heart health through more favorable lipid profiles.

Additionally, monitoring fasting insulin and glucose levels can provide insights into how your body is metabolizing energy, especially as you shift to a fat-based metabolism. Lower fasting insulin and improved insulin sensitivity are markers of metabolic health, and many carnivores find that these markers significantly improve over time, reducing their risk of developing type 2 diabetes or other metabolic disorders.

Other key health markers include C-reactive protein (CRP) and homocysteine, both of which are indicators of inflammation in the body. Lower levels of inflammation are often reported by those on a carnivore diet, as the removal of processed foods, seed oils, and excess carbohydrates can reduce chronic inflammation. Regular tracking allows you to see these improvements in real time, giving you the confidence that this way of eating is benefiting your long-term health.

Longevity Studies and Insights: How Carnivore Dieters Fare Long-Term

When considering any dietary approach for the long term, it is natural to ask, "Will this way of eating support longevity?" While large-scale, long-term studies on the carnivore diet specifically are still emerging, insights can be drawn from related diets that emphasize animal-based nutrition. Research on ketogenic diets, low-carb diets, and ancestral diets has shown positive correlations with longevity, particularly in reducing the risk of chronic diseases like heart disease, diabetes, and neurodegenerative disorders.

One of the most compelling arguments for the carnivore diet's longevity benefits is its impact on metabolic health. By stabilizing blood sugar levels and reducing insulin resistance, the carnivore diet lowers the risk of metabolic syndrome, a condition closely tied to premature aging and reduced lifespan. Those who remain metabolically flexible—able to efficiently use fat for fuel—tend to experience fewer energy crashes, less inflammation, and better overall health as they age.

In addition to metabolic health, the carnivore diet supports longevity through the preservation of muscle mass, which is critical for aging gracefully. As we grow older, muscle mass naturally declines, a process known as sarcopenia. However, diets high in protein, especially from animal sources, are shown to slow this process. By consuming adequate amounts of high-quality protein, carnivore dieters support muscle maintenance, which not only contributes to strength and mobility in later years but also supports metabolic health and insulin sensitivity.

Moreover, the carnivore diet's focus on whole, nutrient-dense foods reduces the consumption of anti-nutrients found in many plants, which can interfere with the absorption of essential minerals. This emphasis on nutrient bioavailability can lead to better bone health, improved cognitive function, and a stronger immune system, all of which are key factors in living a long and vibrant life.

Adjusting the Diet Over Time: When and How to Modify Based on Your Changing Needs
The carnivore diet is not a one-size-fits-all approach. While the foundational principles remain the same—emphasizing animal-based foods—there is flexibility in how the diet can be adapted to meet your needs over time. As you age or as your lifestyle changes, it's important to recognize when and how to make adjustments.

For instance, as you move through different phases of life, your protein needs may fluctuate. Athletes or those focused on building muscle may need more protein than someone who is focused on maintaining their weight. If you are dealing with stress, illness, or recovery from injury, adjusting your fat intake to ensure you are getting adequate energy can be beneficial. The carnivore diet can also be modified to include certain low-carb plants, like avocados or olives, if your body signals a need for additional micronutrients or variety.

Tracking how your body responds to these changes is key. Adjusting the diet does not mean straying from its principles but rather customizing it to ensure that it continues to serve your health and well-being. Listen to your body's signals, and be open to tweaking your approach as necessary, whether that means increasing fat intake during periods of intense exercise or experimenting with different types of animal proteins to see which ones make you feel your best.

Dealing with Plateaus

Why Plateaus Happen: Understanding the Body's Adaptation Process

One of the most frustrating challenges on any long-term diet is hitting a plateau. Whether you're trying to lose weight, gain muscle, or maintain optimal health, there may come a time when progress slows, or stalls completely. Understanding why plateaus happen is the first step in overcoming them.

Plateaus are a natural part of the body's adaptation process. As you lose weight or change your body composition, your body adjusts to its new energy needs. This is often why weight loss may slow down after an initial period of rapid results. Metabolism shifts, and your body becomes more efficient at using the energy it receives, which can make further fat loss or muscle gain more difficult.

For those following the carnivore diet, plateaus may also occur due to a lack of variety in the types of proteins and fats consumed. While the simplicity of the diet is one of its strengths, it can sometimes lead to stagnation if you're not diversifying your food choices. Additionally, factors like stress, sleep quality, and physical activity levels can all impact progress, and these factors should be considered when addressing a plateau.

Breaking Through Plateaus: Strategies to Reignite Fat Loss or Muscle Gain

Breaking through a plateau requires a combination of dietary adjustments and lifestyle changes. One strategy for reigniting fat loss is to experiment with intermittent fasting or time-restricted eating. By narrowing your eating window and allowing your body to spend more time in a fasted state, you can encourage the burning of stored fat for fuel. Many carnivore dieters find success with a 16:8 fasting schedule, where they fast for 16 hours and eat during an 8-hour window.

Another approach is to cycle your macronutrients. If you've been consistently eating a high-protein, moderate-fat carnivore diet, try increasing your fat intake for a period to see if it helps break the plateau. Fat is a more efficient source of energy on a ketogenic or carnivore diet, and increasing your fat intake may help stimulate further fat loss by encouraging deeper ketosis.

For those focused on muscle gain, increasing the variety of proteins can be beneficial. Different animal proteins contain varying levels of amino acids, which are essential for muscle repair and growth. Adding more collagen-rich foods, like bone broth and oxtail, can support joint health and recovery, while leaner cuts of meat may provide the additional protein necessary for muscle synthesis.

Finally, consider the role of physical activity in breaking through a plateau. Strength training, in particular, is a powerful tool for both fat loss and muscle gain. By increasing your lean muscle mass, you'll naturally boost your metabolism, making it easier to continue progressing toward your health goals.

Staying Motivated Long-Term: Tapping into Deeper Purpose and Commitment

When the initial excitement of a new diet fades, and progress slows, staying motivated can be a challenge. However, long-term success on the carnivore diet requires a deeper sense of purpose and commitment. It's essential to connect with why you started this journey in the first place. Whether your goal is improved health, weight loss, or simply feeling better in your body, keeping that vision front and center can help you stay focused when the going gets tough.

A powerful strategy for maintaining motivation is to celebrate small victories along the way. Rather than focusing solely on weight or body composition, pay attention to other markers of success, such as increased energy levels, clearer skin, or improved mental clarity. These are all signs that the diet is working, even if the scale isn't moving as quickly as you'd like.

Additionally, surrounding yourself with a supportive community can be incredibly motivating. Connecting with others who are following the carnivore diet, whether through online forums, social media, or local meetups, can provide the encouragement and accountability needed to stay on track. Sharing your successes and challenges with like-minded individuals creates a sense of camaraderie and can help you push through difficult times.

Final Words on Lifestyle Integration

Balancing Carnivore with Other Life Goals: Career, Family, and Beyond

The carnivore diet, like any lifestyle change, must be balanced with other life goals. It is important to recognize that while the carnivore diet can bring profound benefits, it should seamlessly integrate with your broader life ambitions, including career, family, and personal growth. For many, a rigid focus on dietary choices can lead to unnecessary stress, especially when it feels like it clashes with the demands of daily life. However, when approached with flexibility and understanding, the carnivore diet can enhance your overall well-being and provide the energy and clarity needed to achieve your broader aspirations.

If you're someone with a demanding career, it's crucial to structure your meals in a way that fits into your work schedule without feeling burdensome. Batch cooking, for instance, allows you to prepare larger portions of nutrient-dense meals that can be easily reheated throughout the week. This approach not only saves time but also ensures that you always have access to high-quality food, reducing the temptation to reach for unhealthy snacks or meals when you're under pressure.

For those with families, especially children, finding balance means respecting that not everyone may follow the same eating patterns. Mealtime doesn't have to be complicated. You can enjoy your carnivore meals while still preparing other foods for family members who follow different diets. In fact, leading by example—showing your family that nourishing your body with whole, unprocessed foods improves your mood, energy, and focus—can inspire them to make healthier choices as well.

The key to long-term success is flexibility. There will be times when your diet may need to accommodate social events, travel, or holidays. In these moments, rather than seeing carnivore as restrictive, view it as a framework that supports your goals. By focusing on high-quality proteins, even at a restaurant or when visiting friends, you can continue to feel aligned with your values without drawing unnecessary attention to your dietary choices.

Building a Sustainable, Enjoyable Routine

Sustainability is at the heart of long-term success on the carnivore diet. The goal is to create a routine that is not only health-promoting but also enjoyable. Without enjoyment, even the best diets can feel like a chore. The carnivore diet offers a unique opportunity in this regard because it simplifies the decision-making process around food. When your options are streamlined, it's easier to focus on quality and flavor rather than constantly worrying about what to eat.

One way to build an enjoyable routine is to experiment with different cooking methods. Roasting, grilling, and slow-cooking can all bring out different flavors in meats, and incorporating various cuts of meat can add variety to your meals. It's easy to fall into a pattern of eating the same foods repeatedly, but by being intentional about trying new recipes or cuts, you can keep your meals exciting and satisfying.

Additionally, take the time to develop rituals around food that you enjoy. For some, this might mean creating a weekly steak night where you prepare a special cut of meat and savor it with your family or friends. Others may find joy in crafting the perfect carnivore coffee or indulging in rich, homemade bone broth as part of their morning routine. These rituals elevate the daily act of eating into something more meaningful, creating a deeper connection to the food and its benefits.

Another critical component of sustainability is recognizing when to adjust your routine based on your body's feedback. Some days, you may need more food if you've had a particularly active day. Other times, intermittent fasting may feel more natural. The beauty of the carnivore diet is that it allows for intuitive eating—eating when you're hungry and stopping when you're full. By listening to your body's signals, you'll develop a routine that feels natural and sustainable for the long term.

Embracing a Lifelong Journey: How to Make the Carnivore Diet a Sustainable and Fulfilling Part of Your Life

Ultimately, the carnivore diet is not a short-term fix but a lifelong journey of health and vitality. Like any long-term commitment, there will be highs and lows, but with the right mindset, it can become a deeply fulfilling part of your life. Success comes from viewing this journey not as a set of rigid rules but as a dynamic, evolving process that adapts to your needs.

As you continue on this path, it's essential to reflect on the positive changes you've experienced—whether it's improved energy, better mental clarity, or enhanced physical health. These benefits are not fleeting; they are the result of consistent choices that support your body's natural ability to thrive. Each day on the carnivore diet is a step toward greater health, and by staying committed, you are investing in your future.

One of the most empowering aspects of the carnivore diet is that it encourages self-reliance. As you become more attuned to your body's needs, you'll find that you don't need to rely on external advice or trends to guide your choices. You'll know intuitively what foods make you feel your best and how to adjust your diet based on how you feel. This sense of control over your health is incredibly empowering and can spill over into other areas of your life, fostering a sense of confidence and resilience.

Finally, embrace the community that comes with following a carnivore lifestyle. There are countless individuals around the world who have found success and joy in this way of eating, and connecting with them can provide motivation and support as you continue on your journey. Whether through social media, online forums, or local groups, the carnivore community is a resource for sharing recipes, experiences, and advice.

By embracing the carnivore diet as a lifelong journey rather than a temporary solution, you'll create a relationship with food that is both sustainable and fulfilling. The ultimate goal is to live a life of health, vitality, and enjoyment, free from the constant struggles many face around food and diet. This journey is about more than just what you eat—it's about how you feel, how you move through the world, and how you live your life.

In the end, sustaining long-term success on the carnivore diet requires a combination of practical strategies, personal insight, and a deep connection to your health and well-being. By monitoring your progress, overcoming challenges, and integrating this way of eating into your broader life goals, you'll not only thrive in the short term but also enjoy a lifetime of health and vitality. This is the power of the carnivore diet: a path to enduring success that nourishes both body and mind, allowing you to live your best life, every day.

AUTHOR'S FINAL NOTE

As I sit here reflecting on the journey that led to the creation of this book, Carnivore Diet for Longevity & Vitality: Unlock the Secrets to Optimal Health, Mental Clarity, and Emotional Wellness, I am reminded of the many questions that propelled me into the world of nutrition and well-being. Like many of you, I've experienced moments of confusion in a world overflowing with dietary advice, often contradictory and overwhelming. The sheer number of diets, trends, and fads seemed to pull in every direction, promising results but rarely delivering on all fronts—health, clarity, and a sense of overall balance.

This book was born out of a desire to cut through the noise. I wanted to provide a roadmap to a lifestyle that not only focuses on health but on thriving—physically, mentally, and emotionally. The carnivore diet, though initially met with skepticism by many, has proven to be transformative for countless individuals. Its simplicity, rooted in ancestral wisdom and supported by modern science, has offered a path to those seeking clarity amidst the clutter. My goal in writing this book was to share these profound benefits with you, not as an abstract concept but as a practical, achievable reality that you can integrate into your daily life.

The Aim of This Book

At its core, Carnivore Diet for Longevity & Vitality is not just about what you eat. Yes, it's about food, but it's also about the journey toward self-awareness, self-improvement, and self-empowerment. The carnivore diet is a tool, a powerful one, that gives you control over your health. This book aims to empower you with knowledge so that you can make informed choices—not just about the diet but about how you live your life, manage your stress, and enhance your mental and emotional well-being.

I wanted to challenge the misconceptions around eating animal-based foods and debunk the myths that have led so many to fear fat, shun cholesterol, or overcomplicate their nutritional lives. This book is designed to be both an educational tool and a practical guide, providing you with the information, support, and tools to make real, lasting changes in your life.

If you've felt lost or uncertain in your quest for better health, I hope this book has provided clarity. If you've struggled with conflicting advice and endless debates over the "right" way to eat, I hope you find peace in knowing that there is a path that works for many—a path that is intuitive, natural, and deeply rooted in our evolutionary history. My aim has been to show you that health doesn't have to be complicated. It can be simple, effective, and sustainable.

The Benefits You Can Expect

When you embark on the carnivore diet, you'll begin to experience changes not just in how you look, but in how you feel—both mentally and emotionally. For some, the initial benefits are physical: weight loss, improved energy, and fewer digestive issues. But the longer you follow this path, the more you'll notice deeper, more profound changes.

Your mind will sharpen, free from the fog that many of us have accepted as part of daily life. Your mood will stabilize, your sense of well-being will grow, and you'll find a mental clarity that you may not have known was possible. Emotionally, the carnivore diet can help you build resilience, regulate your mood, and boost your self-confidence. There is something empowering about aligning your diet with your body's needs, knowing that you are giving it the fuel it was designed to thrive on.

And then there's longevity—the ultimate goal for many. The carnivore diet is not about short-term fixes or temporary results. It's about creating a foundation for long-term health. By prioritizing nutrient-dense, bioavailable foods that support muscle mass, bone strength, metabolic health, and cognitive function, you're giving yourself the best possible chance at a long, vibrant life.

Why This Book Matters

You might ask, "Why focus on the carnivore diet?" There are certainly many other diets and approaches out there. But what sets the carnivore diet apart is its simplicity and its alignment with our biology. We are, at our core, omnivorous beings who have evolved to thrive on a diet rich in animal foods. The modern world has led many of us astray, filling our plates with processed, nutrient-poor foods that don't nourish our bodies the way they should. This diet strips all of that away and brings us back to basics.

I'm not here to argue that the carnivore diet is for everyone, but I do believe that it can offer profound benefits to those who feel lost in the sea of dietary advice. It is especially beneficial for those who have struggled with metabolic issues, inflammation, digestive problems, and even mental health challenges. There's a growing body of evidence that suggests the carnivore diet can help people regain control of their health, and it's my hope that this book has made that case convincingly.

In this book, I've outlined the various aspects of the carnivore diet, from its historical roots to its modern applications. I've discussed the health benefits, the science behind it, and provided you with practical advice on how to implement it in your life. Whether you're looking to lose weight, boost your energy, or simply feel better, I hope you'll find the tools you need within these pages.

A Personal Journey

Writing this book has been as much a personal journey as it has been a professional one. In researching and writing about the carnivore diet, I've deepened my understanding of nutrition, health, and well-being. I've had the privilege of connecting with countless individuals who have experienced life-changing transformations through this way of eating. Their stories have inspired me and reaffirmed the importance of sharing this knowledge with as many people as possible.

This journey has also been about challenging my own beliefs. I, too, was once skeptical of a diet that seemed so far removed from the conventional wisdom we've been taught for decades. But the more I learned, the more I realized that so much of what we've been told about health, nutrition, and disease prevention has been flawed. The carnivore diet opened my eyes to a new way of thinking about food and health, and I hope it has done the same for you.

Your Journey Moving Forward

Now, as you prepare to take your next steps, I encourage you to embrace this journey with an open mind and a commitment to your health. Like any change, adopting the carnivore diet will come with its challenges, but the rewards are well worth it. You might face skepticism from friends or family, and there will be days when it feels difficult. But remember that you are in control of your health and your body. You are the one who gets to decide what works best for you.

Use the tools provided in this book—whether it's the meal plans, recipes, or practical advice—as a foundation for your journey. But don't be afraid to make adjustments based on your own experience. The beauty of the carnivore diet is its flexibility and adaptability. You can make it your own.

Most importantly, be patient with yourself. Lasting change takes time, and health is a lifelong journey. Celebrate your victories, no matter how small, and keep moving forward. As you continue on this path, remember that you are not alone. There is a community of like-minded individuals who have found success on the carnivore diet, and they are here to support you.

Final Thoughts

In closing, I want to express my gratitude to you for taking the time to read this book and for being open to a new way of thinking about food and health. My hope is that the information contained in these pages has not only informed you but has inspired you to take control of your health in a way that feels empowering and sustainable.

This is more than just a diet—it's a lifestyle, a mindset, and a journey toward better health, greater vitality, and a more fulfilling life. Thank you for allowing me to be a part of your journey. I wish you all the best as you move forward, confident in your choices and committed to your well-being.

To your health and happiness,

Julianna Irvin Saladino

ABOUT THE AUTHOR

Julianna Irvin Saladino is a distinguished authority in health and wellness, dedicated to helping individuals reclaim their vitality through evidence-based dietary and lifestyle changes. With a robust background in nutritional science and over a decade of hands-on experience in holistic health, Julianna has established herself as a leading voice in the field, cutting through the clutter of modern dietary advice to deliver clear, actionable strategies that produce real results.

Her career is marked by a steadfast commitment to her readers' well-being. Julianna has successfully guided thousands on their journey to optimal health, helping them overcome chronic fatigue, inflammation, and weight challenges. Her expertise is grounded in both meticulous research and a profound understanding of the psychological and emotional dimensions of dietary transformation.

Julianna's personal health journey, which involved a remarkable transformation through strategic nutrition, deeply influences her writing and coaching. Her experience allows her to offer not only expert knowledge but also empathetic support, acknowledging the complexities and victories inherent in making significant lifestyle changes.

In addition to her role as an author, Julianna is a sought-after speaker and wellness coach, renowned for her ability to translate complex nutritional concepts into practical advice. Her dedication extends beyond her written work; she actively engages with her audience through online communities, workshops, and personalized coaching, providing ongoing support and insights.

Julianna Irvin Saladino's approach transcends conventional dietary advice. Her work is a testament to empowering individuals to lead their best lives, unburdened by modern health challenges. Whether you're embarking on a new dietary path or seeking to deepen your understanding of nutrition, Julianna's expertise offers a guiding light in the quest for enhanced well-being.

Discover More Titles by Julianna Irvin Saladino on Amazon!

If you've enjoyed this book, be sure to explore Julianna's complete collection of works. Whether you're diving into health, fitness, or personal empowerment through nutrition & lifestyle changes, there's a book for you! Start your next adventure today—just head over to my Amazon Author Page to explore more or search my name and see all titles under my name

Did you enjoy reading this book? Check out other amazing titles on Dieting, Food & Nutrition by the author on Amazon

1. THE ALL-IN-ONE 30-DAYS MEAL PLAN & RECIPES CARNIVORE DIET COOKBOOK FOR BEGINNERS & PROS!
2. THE KETO DIET ULTIMATE SUSTAINABLE WEIGHT LOSS & OPTIMAL HEALTH GUIDE FOR BEGINNERS
3. THE ESSENTIAL KETO MEAL PREP DIET COOKBOOK FOR BEGINNERS & PROS, 2024
4. PROVEN QUICK & EASY GLUTEN-FREE VEGAN COOKBOOK FOR BEGINNERS
5. THE IDEAL BEGINNER'S COOKBOOK GUIDE TO A PLANT-BASED DIET
6. THE COMPLETE CODE CARNIVORE COOKBOOK
7. THE COMPLETE CARNIVORE COOKBOOK FOR TEENS & YOUNG ADULTS